医学研究生
综合英语

主 编 王泽阳 吕鹏飞
副主编 陈道胜 袁昌万 冯 颖

编 委（以姓氏拼音为序）

陈道胜 陈建平 冯 颖
吕鹏飞 谢婷婷 袁昌万
弋 倩 王泽阳 赵洪霞

English
for Medical Graduate Students

上海交通大学出版社
SHANGHAI JIAO TONG UNIVERSITY PRESS

内容提要

  本书为医学研究生英语教材,共 8 个单元,每个单元由两大部分组成。第一部分为医学相关主题的精读,配备了词汇、阅读、翻译、讨论、课堂展示等练习,将医学主题与语言学习有机结合起来,更符合医学研究生的英语学习特点。第二部分为促进学生学术发展而设计,包含中文论文摘要翻译和医学英文论文写作。本书兼具专业性和人文性,能满足医学研究生的英语语言学习需求和学术发展需求,适合医学专业研究生使用。

图书在版编目(CIP)数据

  医学研究生综合英语/王泽阳,吕鹏飞主编. —上海:上海交通大学出版社,2022.8
  ISBN 978 - 7 - 313 - 26914 - 0

  Ⅰ.①医… Ⅱ.①王…②吕… Ⅲ.①医学—英语—研究—教材 Ⅳ.①R

  中国版本图书馆 CIP 数据核字(2022)第 129181 号

医学研究生综合英语
YIXUE YANJIUSHENG ZONGHE YINGYU

主　　编:	王泽阳　吕鹏飞			
出版发行:	上海交通大学出版社		地　　址:	上海市番禺路 951 号
邮政编码:	200030		电　　话:	021 - 64071208
印　　制:	上海万卷印刷股份有限公司		经　　销:	全国新华书店
开　　本:	710mm×1000mm　1/16		印　　张:	10
字　　数:	219 千字			
版　　次:	2022 年 8 月第 1 版		印　　次:	2022 年 8 月第 1 次印刷
书　　号:	ISBN 978 - 7 - 313 - 26914 - 0			
定　　价:	42.00 元			

前　言

　　为贯彻《普通高等学校教材管理办法》精神，加快一流专业、一流课程和一流教材建设，川北医学院决定从2021年起资助线上线下混合式教材编写申报立项工作，《医学研究生综合英语》是获得第一批资助的教材之一。

　　本教材注重研究生阶段对专业知识以及人文情怀培养的双重要求，内容上兼具专业性和人文性，能满足医学研究生的英语语言学习需求和学术发展需求。教材注重培养研究生的英语语言实际运用能力和创新思维能力，尤其注重培养跨文化交际能力，以适应"双一流"建设的拔尖创新医学人才的国际化需要。

　　医学研究生英语属于专门用途英语的一个分支，是特定学术语境下的英语教学。教材以医学相关内容为依托开展英语教学，将语言学习与医学专业知识结合起来，将语言作为了解和获取信息的途径而非单纯学习语言本身。通过本教材的学习，我们希望学生能熟练运用英语搜索和阅读专业文献资料，获取最前沿的信息，能用英语归纳和表达专业领域信息，撰写英语学术论文，并能用英语与专业人士顺利进行交流。

　　本教材共8个单元，每个单元分为两大部分，第一部分以一个视频材料引出主题，随后是与该主题相关的精读文本，文本后配备了词汇、阅读、翻译、讨论、课堂展示等练习。词汇练习精选自教学团队及川北医学院近几届研究生共同搜集整理的医学素材语料库。通过该部分练习，学生不但可以学习和巩固词汇表达，还可以提高医学题材文本的阅读水平，熟悉医学学术写作，起到以点带面的作用。阅读和翻译练习结合精读文本主题，略有延伸，凸显了语言的实际运用。讨论与课堂展示以问题的形式激发学生的思考，锻炼学生的口头表达能力。第二部分为学术发展，由医学小论文摘要的汉英翻译和医学论文写作方法介绍两部分组成。其中，用于汉英

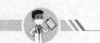

翻译的摘要选自与单元主题相关的中文期刊论文,通过该部分内容学习和练习,让学生掌握论文摘要翻译的方法和技巧,以便顺利完成自己论文摘要的英文翻译。医学论文写作方法部分主要面向有发表英文期刊论文需求的学生,每个章节分别介绍了英文论文写作的一个方面,以期起到领路的作用。

本教材主要有以下三个方面的特点:

(1)三个层级。为了满足不同语言基础学生对语言学习的需求,教材各单元的选材都分为三个层级,即大众级、科普级和学术级。大众级选材主要是医学主题的报道材料,作为单元学习的基础,可供语言基础一般的学生重点学习;科普级在难度上有所提升,需要具备一定专业知识才能听懂、读懂,供绝大部分学生学习;学术级主要节选自学术论文和学术著作,助力学术研究和交流。

(2)中外兼收。每个单元所选材料均纳入中国学者的作品或讲述中国故事的外籍学者作品,充分融入中国元素和中国经验。这样的目的是适应中国学者在国际学术界影响力不断提升的现实,也能更好实现研究生英语课程思政的全覆盖。同时可以通过中国人在国际社会的经验,更加直接地影响和启发中国的在读研究生。

(3)线上线下立体资源。研究生英语的一大作用是帮助学生了解和获取领域最前沿的信息,而纸质教材很难做到实时更新,并不能很好地实现这一功能。医学知识更新速度快,纸质教材提供的信息只是冰山一角。因此,除了纸质版精选材料之外,教材还结合线上学习平台,持续更新和丰富教学资源,为学生提供更多、更新的学习参考资料。获取本书 Lead-in 部分的音视频及 Further Readings 部分的文章,请在"交大外语"微信公众号后台留言。

本教材从构思到立项,从编写到出版都得到了川北医学院教务处、研究生处和外国语言文化系的大力支持和资助。上海交通大学出版社的编辑们也在编写和出版过程中给予了大力支持。编写过程中,我们也得到了许多外语界同行和医学专家的关心和帮助,他们给予了我们许多建设性的意见和建议,在此一并表示衷心的感谢和敬意。

由于编者学识有限,书中难免存在不足或疏漏之处,恳请广大同行专家和读者不吝赐教,以期再版时修正和完善。

编者

2022 年 3 月于果城嘉陵江畔

目　　录

Unit 1

Public Health Care

Lead-in : Sunshine on the Road

(Task 1) *Watch the video and answer the following questions, and then exchange your answers with your classmates.*

1. What is happening in Tongguanyi town, Chongqing in southwest China according to the video?

   _____

   _____

2. What does the rural project in China supported by the World Bank aim to do according to the video?

   _____

   _____

(Task 2) *Watch the video again and fill the following gaps. Make sure the word(s) you fill in is(are) both grammatically and semantically acceptable.*

In Tongguanyi town, Chongqing in southwest China, an innovative pilot program is underway to deliver health services to people. It's coming from the special team of doctors set up by the township health center of Tongguanyi. (1) _____ who now pay visits to patients in remote villages, especially (2) _____.

In China, (3) _____ typically go to big hospitals in cities. Family doctors are scarce. And for rural residents, transport to city hospitals can be

(4) _____ , but no more for 70-year-old Chen Guangming, from Doushita village.

Today, Chen should have another (5) _____ , her doctors are already (6) _____ . It rained earlier and the road is wet and slippery. But it's no problem for these doctors who bike to see their patients (7) _____ . Four of them here are to visit Chen and her families. On their backs is the team's name (8) _____ with the aim of bringing rural families' health care that's as warm and accessible as sunshine. They are part of many innovations of the World Bank that supported rural health projects, which is working to bridge the gap between rural and urban health services. It takes (9) _____ for the doctors to arrive at Chen's house.

As they leave, the doctors give (10) _____ to Chen to take her pills. The next morning, the doctors are back on the road.

Part I   Intensive Reading

The Development and Reform of Public Health Care in China
(1949 – 2019)
By Li Wang, Zhihao Wang, et al.

1 China's public health has developed for 7 decades since the founding of the People's Republic of China(P. R. C.). Looking back, there was unique Chinese wisdom and remarkable achievements as well as twists and turns on the journey of reform. In the past 70 years, China has made great strides in providing equitable and accessible public health services to its citizens, and built up a well-established service delivery system. As a result, the health status of Chinese people has been enhanced significantly since 1949, and public health has contributed 77.9% to the increase of life expectancy.

2 In early times, China's success in controlling infectious diseases can be attributed in a large part to the public health system in four aspects. ①The prevention-first and preemptive approach. During that period, guidelines and policies, resource allocation, as well as organizational structure of the health sector centered around prevention and control of infectious diseases. That was aligned with the spectrum of disease at that time, therefore led to outstanding outcomes. ②Flexible structure of the system. For example, to fill the huge gap of health workforce at that time, a great amount of barefoot doctors came to the fore. They were both farmers and PHC

(Primary Health Care) personnel. Their income came from their farming work and payment from village collective economy for their public health services. Besides, their good knowledge on local environment and local people in the catchment was helpful to provide effective public health services. Thus, they made remarkable contribution to the progress in China's public health. ③ The three-tiered service delivery network, and collaboration within the network and with non-health sectors. The three levels were complementary and coordinated in prevention, treatment and other care. Patriotic Health Campaign Committee was a typical example of the multi-agency collaboration. ④ Innovative mechanism of mass mobilization and society participation. For instance, besides its administrative system to coordinate different agencies, the Patriotic Health Campaign established some civil societies at grassroots level so that every household was mobilized to implement the Campaign and the whole society participated effectively.

3 China's market-oriented financing reforms initiated in the late 1970s created both opportunities and challenges for the health system. On the one hand, it mobilized more resources from health service users and improved working conditions. On the other hand, it drastically reduced government spending on health. At that time, more and more public health service providers tended to provide profitable charged services including outpatient and inpatient services, but ignored the fact that the public health system in rural areas was on the brink of collapse then, which led to the decline of epidemic prevention and control capacity.

4 Despite twists and turns, China's public health system has always been resilient. System resilience is defined as "the capacity of a system to absorb disturbance and reorganize while undergoing change so as to still retain essentially the same function, structure, identity, and feedback". The public health system in China was impacted badly by the market-oriented healthcare reform in the 1980s, but got back to the right track after the SARS outbreak. In many countries, public health crisis is an external driver to improve their system.

5 The renewed attention to public health in China was triggered by the SARS outbreak. But the sustained progress is driven by the government's commitment to social development and people's livelihoods, and backed by robust economic growth and strong government leadership. After SARS crisis, government's role and responsibilities in the health sector were further clarified, and the growth rate of government spending on health was required to be higher than the growth rate of government spending. For example, per capita expenditure on National Basic Public Health Service Program increased from 15 yuan in 2009 to 55 yuan in 2018. This period also registered rapid economic growth and great improvement of peoples' living standard in China.

6 Moreover, rapid development of China's health sector is also associated with the strong leadership of the government. Most major strategies and guidelines in health sector were proposed at CPC Congress, and their implementation also followed the "public policy implementation mechanism with Chinese characteristics under the leadership of the CPC". Prasenjit Duara, a famous American Sinologist, pointed out that China's success to much degree lies in the strong party organization, which is deeply rooted in Chinese urban and rural areas. The party and the state have sufficient power of mobilization. In a word, it is fair to say that, from the development of the public health emergency system from scratch, to the rapid expansion of the traditional disease prevention and control system and health supervision system, this period was not only the transition trajectory of China's rural health system, but also the golden time for the development and construction of China's public health institutions.

7 In the 2010s, the Chinese government pays unprecedented attention to the health sector, presses ahead with new round of healthcare reform, and formulates the strategies of "Healthy China" and "no well-off society without a healthy population". Among BRICs countries, China registers the most rapid development in health system and is the most significant member in terms of global outreach. China's share of nominal total health expenditure (THE) composition in BRICs rose from 29% in 1993 to 52% in 2012, gradually achieving a dominant position from year to year, and representing the largest share of total THE of BRICs. All of these bring a new wave of opportunities to public health in China. At this stage, the goal is to make the system more equitable and people-centered. The National Basic Public Health Service Program (NBPHSP) remains the priority. It is designed to provide rural and urban residents with free basic public health services covering total population throughout the whole life cycle, which increases the accessibility and affordability of basic public health services. Compared with Brazil and India, rural Chinese have much higher gains in equity of access to health care in China, although all BRICs countries have very uneven population distribution with exceptionally large rural areas. However, there are challenges in NBPHSP implementation, including concerns on the quality of services, the package that is not updated timely, poor integration of the system and inadequate human resources.

8 In China, quality concerns to a large extent are attributable to insufficient per capita health expenditure. BRICs' joint share of global health spending is far less than that of OECD (Organization for Economic Co-operation and Development). Among BRICs members, per capita health expenditure in Russia and Brazil exceeds that in

China three times and more than twice respectively, which may indicate that Chinese health reform still has a long way to go. However, some OECD countries suffer from surge in health expenditure with few marginal health gains. China needs to avoid it, although its per capita health spending is still relatively low.

9 Integration of health systems is the direction of future efforts in the world. The UN Sustainable Development Goals (SDGs) highlights organic connections and systematic approach among a variety of health factors, and enhancing overall health system is more important in the SDG era. However, China's public health service system is still facing insufficient integration problems such as poor service items integration, insufficient intersetoral actions, isolated IT system and so on. The effectiveness of cooperation mechanisms on health issues among different sectors depends heavily on factors such as organizational structure, management, culture, and trust. We argue that ever effective coordinate mechanisms such as the Patriotic Health Campaign Committee in China can be further applied to cope with emerging public health challenges such as ageing and NCDs.

10 The lack of health human resources at the grass-roots level, especially in rural areas, is an important problem that China and other emerging developing countries are facing. Doctors and nurses are reluctant to be employed by primary health facilities most of which are located in the countryside. It is an obstacle to develop sufficient and effective public health workforce.

11 From a global perspective, most countries are in the transformation of public health landscape, due to common emerging challenges. The development and reform of public health in China needs to be further deepened. Firstly, accelerated aeging population is placing a number of countries in a substantial disadvantage position in healthcare reforms. Developing countries are experiencing much more rapid aeging process than rich countries, and China is the fastest one in the upcoming decades. This is a serious potential risk to the financial sustainability of China's health sector in a broader sense. Furthermore, lower fertility willingness may exacerbate the risk. Secondly, NCDs are recognized as the key health challenge worldwide, and are already China's number one health threat. Unlike infectious diseases which have relatively short acute phase and take less time to cure, NCDs will bring massive and long-term burden for both patients and the society. Moreover, the prevalence of NCDs among the elderly is disproportionately high, and some of them often have more than one NCD. Emerging NCDs burden coupled with aeging population means that sustainability challenge in public health system will be very serious, even in the richest OECD countries. Thirdly, social and economic transformation have accelerated urbanization and changes in life style, leading to many risk factors such as obesity, sedentary lifestyles, stress, tobacco/ alcohol/other substances abuse, and exposure to pollution. The incidence of NCDs is also rising due to these individual or environmental factors. Fourthly, globalization accelerates the spread of infectious diseases, imposing challenges to public health. Many countries including China face the dual burden of NCDs and infectious diseases at the same time.

12 In a nutshell, the evolution and reform of China's public health is based on its national condition. During the process, China accumulates rich experience but also faces many common worldwide challenges which may be even more pronounced in China.

13 However, it is expected that government's continuous attention to the health sector and its stable macro environment will be greatly helpful to address those challenges. Getting this development and reform right is important to China's social and economic development in future, and we believe that China's experience in public health may provide many lessons for other countries.

Words and Expressions

equitable /ˈekwɪtəbl/ *adj.*　　fair and impartial

accessible /əkˈsesɪbl/ *adj.*　　(of a place) able to be reached or entered

enhance /ɪnˈhɑːns/ *v.*　　to intensify, increase, or further improve the quality, value, or extent of

remarkable /rɪˈmɑːkəbl/ *adj.*　　worthy of attention; striking

mobilize /ˈməʊbəlaɪz/ *v.*　　(of a country or its government) to prepare and organize (troops) for active service

initiate /ɪˈnɪʃɪeɪt/ *v.*　　cause (a process or action) to begin

resilient /rɪˈzɪliənt/ *adj.*　　able to recoil or spring back into shape after bending, stretching, or being compressed

retain /rɪˈteɪn/ *v.*　　to continue to have (something); keep possession of

sustain /səˈsteɪn/ *v.*　　to strengthen or support physically or mentally

commitment /kəˈmɪtmənt/ *n.*　　a pledge or undertaking

external /ɪkˈstɜːnəl/ *adj.*　　coming or derived from a source outside the subject affected

expenditure /ɪkˈspendɪtʃə/ *n.*　　the action of spending funds

nominal /ˈnɒmɪnəl/ *adj.*　　(of a role or status) existing in name only

trajectory /trəˈdʒektəri/ *n.*　　the path followed by a projectile flying or an object moving under the action of given forces

unprecedented /ʌnˈpresɪdentɪd/ *adj.*	never done or known before
formulate /ˈfɔːmjʊleɪt/ *v.*	to create or prepare methodically
outreach /ˈaʊtriːtʃ/ *n.*	the extent or length of reaching out
priority /praɪˈɒrəti/ *n.*	the fact or condition of being regarded or treated as more important than others
distribution /ˌdɪstrɪˈbjuːʃn/ *n.*	the action of sharing something out among a number of recipients
marginal /ˈmɑːdʒɪnəl/ *n.*	minor and not important; not central
coordinate /kəʊˈɔːdɪneɪt/ *adj.*	equal in rank or importance
perspective /pəˈspektɪv/ *n.*	a view or prospect
accelerate /əkˈseləreɪt/ *v.*	to increase in rate, amount, or extent
sedentary /ˈsedəntəri/ *adj.*	(of a person) tending to spend much time seated; somewhat inactive
disproportionate /ˌdɪsprəˈpɔːʃənət/ *adj.*	surprising or unreasonable in amount or size, compared with something else
pronounce /prəˈnaʊns/ *v.*	to declare or announce in a formal or solemn way

I. Reading Comprehension

Choose the best answer to each of the following questions.

1. How much has public health contributed to the increase of Chinese people's life expectancy since the founding of the P. R. C.?

   A. About 22.1%.　　B. About 80%.　　C. About 29%.　　D. About 52%.

2. China owe much of its early success in controlling infectious diseases to _____.

   A. the prevention-first and preemptive approach

   B. flexible structure of the system and the three-tiered service delivery network

   C. innovative mechanism of mass mobilization and society participation

   D. All of the above.

3. What is the main reason for the rapid development of public health in China according to Prasenjit Duara, a famous American Sinologist?

   A. China's public health has always been resilient.

   B. The renewed attention to public health in China triggered by the SARS outbreak.

   C. The strong party organization.

   D. The strong leadership of the government.

4. What is the problem China is facing now in public health service system?

   A. Insufficient integration.　　　　B. Organizational structure.

C. Ageing population and NCDs.   D. The direction of future efforts.

5. Which of the following is NOT one of the common challenges to global public health?

A. Accelerated aeging population and NCDs (Non-communicable Diseases).

B. Urbanization and changes in life style accelerated by social and economic transformation leads to many risk factors.

C. The spread of infectious diseases, accelerated by globalization imposes challenges to public health.

D. The lack of health human resources at the grass-roots level, especially in rural areas.

II. Vocabulary

(Task 1) *Fill in the blanks of the following sentences with the words or expressions given in the box below. Change the forms where necessary.*

equitable	accessible	enhance	charge	mobilize
initiate	retain	sustain	external	expenditure
nominal	resilient	formulate	marginal	perspective

1. Everything is easily _____ to the customer, who is left free to browse until assistance is needed.

2. Much confusion exists regarding the tariff payable by the medical aid funds and the amount _____ by the various service providers or institutions.

3. You're never going to be able to activate or _____ a group of workers if you're campaigning for something that they don't care about.

4. We have the meals and snacks that will _____ our mental and physical stamina from dawn to dusk.

5. To be negotiable and have legitimacy, commitments generally need to be perceived to be reasonably fair and _____.

6. The report proposed that the authority _____ a procurement process to enable anyone to put forward any technologies for waste disposal.

7. It is time to think, plan and _____ a strong antibiotic policy to address the burgeoning hospital infection.

8. The government plays a _____ role in dictating policy because it cannot monitor local fisheries or enforce fisheries regulations.

9. It may be sensible to use it to pay for a major home repair or improvement that will

_____ the quality of your life.

10. The belief that girls are more _____ to environmental factors than boys was thus not supported.

11. Conductors, too, can _____ their musical powers long after physical vigor has departed.

12. The antigen was more abundant in the zone adjacent to the plasma membrane than in the zone closer to the _____ wall surface.

13. This gives a panoramic _____ of the church as it spans across time and space.

14. This in turn results in inefficient administration and inefficient _____ of available funds.

15. In 1914, the submarine was seen as a weapon of _____ importance, in other words, submarines did not play a major role then.

Task 2　*Under each of the following boxes there are several groups of sentences. In each group, a common word or expression is missing. Find it out from the corresponding box according to the meaning and structure of the sentences. The forms of the words and expressions may change in the sentences.*

outreach	trajectory	distribution	unprecedented

Group 1

1. Despite the importance of this objective, other significant health problems may persist or become apparent later in the course of the cancer _____.

2. At any time, a number of different versions of the patient can be in circulation with information pertinent to healthcare _____ management distributed in time and space.

3. Generated initially through the nursing admission process, _____ narratives are continuously reviewed and revised in response to the changes in a patient care.
Answer: _____

Group 2

1. A novel concept is to emulate the dose _____ achieved by intracavitary brachytherapy by external-beam techniques such as stereotactic radiosurgery.

2. It is a typical member of the IQGAP protein family and likely to be an integral part of the function of these proteins, but its wider _____ in the proteome remains to be determined.

3. Cytoplasmic _____ and degradation also contributed to the evolution of alternative splicing.

Answer: _____

Group 3

1. In the wake of an _____ number of U. S. Food and Drug Administration approvals for cancer immunotherapy agents, particularly immune checkpoint inhibitors, the field is poised for further advancement.

2. Notwithstanding _____ volume of investigations on the H. pylori infection worldwide, its effective eradication remains as a dilemma.

3. This symposium: Building Bridges Through Science and Global Health, was followed by an _____ visit by the participating Cuban scientists to the NIH in Bethesda, Maryland.

Answer: _____

Group 4

1. The Research and Development Institute has launched a media-based hepatitis B education and _____ campaign.

2. We completed a controlled trial of a community _____ intervention to promote recognition and receipt of CBEs, mammograms and Pap smears among women.

3. _____ efforts entailed development and distribution of Vietnamese-language health education materials that are appropriate to the culture and education of these recently emigrated women.

Answer: _____

sedentary	disproportionately	commitment	accelerate

Group 5

1. While some will likely be achievable without undue effort, others will require systematic restructuring of the care provided to cancer survivors, such as recommendations to improve opportunities in survivorship research, will require a significant _____ from the health care community, including funding agencies invested in advancing cancer care.

2. The organization benefits from the improved working atmosphere and the active _____ of its practitioners, as well as from the positive image and success projected to the outside world.

3. They should also have congruent philosophies and values and a _____ to collaboration and mutual cooperation as well.

Answer: _____

Group 6

1. Researchers cited several mechanisms of age-related deterioration of intervertebral discs, but they acknowledged that activities and agents that _____ degeneration remain speculative.

2. We found that increased CIMT was significantly correlated with inflammatory measures, suggesting that systemic inflammation in AS may _____ the atherosclerotic process.

3. Biomarker-based approaches as well as fixed randomization alternatives, represent major advances in trial design that should _____ identification of predictive biomarkers for novel therapeutics.

Answer: _____

Group 7

1. Endurance exercise training is associated with lower levels of stiffness in central arteries, which suggests that regular exercise may be able to delay or prevent age-related increases in arterial stiffness. A single bout of aerobic exercise can improve endothelial function in _____ and physically active individuals.

2. A cross-sectional study by Cooks and colleagues showed that rowing, which has both aerobic and resistance exercise components, has an overall positive effect on arterial stiffness compared with _____ controls.

3. Individual differences in fitness level, physical ability, and trainability may have also influenced study outcomes despite all participants being recruited as _____ or only participating in low levels of activity.

Answer: _____

Group 8

1. While Vietnamese women have a low incidence of breast cancer, they have a _____ high incidence of cervical cancer compared to women in the general population.

2. The presence of a fragility fracture puts a patient at a _____ higher risk of another fragility fracture.

3. In some contexts translational mobilization work will be evenly distributed between actors, in others, it might fall _____ to particular occupational groups or be accomplished primarily through technologies.

Answer: _____

III. Cloze

Fill in each of the following blanks with the most appropriate word from each of the four choices given.

In October 2016, President Xi Jinping announced the Healthy China (HC 2030) blueprint, a bold declaration that made public health a __1__ for all future economic and social development.

The HC 2030 blueprint, __2__ in Beijing by the Chinese government, includes 29 chapters __3__ public health services, environment management, the Chinese medical industry, and food and drug safety. The HC 2030 blueprint has been established as a national __4__ and sets a goal of enabling everyone to be involved in health, share health, and be __5__ for health. There are five specific goals to improve the level of health nationwide, control major risk factors, increase the capacity of the health service, enlarge the scale of the health industry, and perfect the health service system. The blueprint is based on four core __6__, that is, health priority, reform and __7__, scientific development, and justice and equity, and outlines 13 core indicators to be reported in 2020 and 2030.

Health is the __8__ prerequisite for the overall well-being of people as well as the foundation of economic and social development. The Program for a Healthy China 2030 __9__ and approved by the Political Bureau of the CPC Central Committee has set an action plan for the construction of a healthy China in the next 15 years. With a profound understanding of the great strategic significance of a healthy China, we need to make an effort from the __10__ of constructing a society that is well off in all aspects of life, foster a new engine for economic and social development, improve structural reform of the medical supply side, enhance national well-being and social stability, __11__ global healthy governance, and fulfill the __12__ that China has made to the international community.

We need to not only have a clear understanding of the progress China has made in medical and health services, but also face the challenges in constructing a healthy China. After years of ongoing efforts, a basic national health insurance system has been completed, and __13__ progress has been made in the reform of the medical health care system. As a result, improvement in health care is moving forward __14__; a healthy environment in relation to the atmosphere and water quality has been achieved to some extent. In the meantime, as a result of industrialization and __15__, ageing of the population, continuous changes in disease spectra, ecological conditions, and people's lifestyles, there are still some weak areas to be improved with regard to the development of health undertakings.

1. A. condition   B. precondition   C. situation   D. environment

2. A. generalized   B. utilized   C. employed   D. released

3. A. covering   B. covered   C. discovered   D. recovered

4. A. tactics   B. strategy   C. conspiracy   D. stigma

5. A. responsive   B. irresponsible

     C. responsible   D. comprehensible

6. A. principals   B. prerequisite   C. recognition   D. principles

7. A. innovation   B. innovative   C. novelty   D. inspiration

8. A. dispensable   B. indispensable

     C. indistinguishable   D. distinguishable

9. A. viewed   B. visualized   C. reviewed   D. virtualized

10. A. perspective   B. prospective   C. perception   D. reception

11. A. propose   B. propel   C. propaganda   D. process

12. A. committee   B. commitment   C. commission   D. contemplation

13. A. luxurious   B. extravagant   C. remarkable   D. simultaneous

14. A. slimly   B. sturdily   C. stoutly   D. swiftly

15. A. urbanization   B. ruralization

     C. industrialization   D. modernization

IV. Discussion and Presentation

Answer the following questions on the basis of your reading.

1. The saying "Trade life for money when young and trade money for life when aged" to some extent reflects people's conception of healthcare and money. What's your comment on this statement?

2. How much do you know about the current situation of rural health care in China?

3. In your opinion, what are the biggest health care problems in China nowadays?

V. Translation

Translate the following sentences into English.

1. 如今,人们对公共卫生的需求已经从"疾病防控"转向"健康促进"。

_____

_____

2. 许多人认为私立医院资源有限,医生水平不如公立医院,纯粹是为了牟利。

_____

_____

3. 打击黄牛党、减轻过分拥挤的公立医院的负担,其措施包括推广医疗应用、增加私立医院数量。

_____

_____

4. 为了解决超负荷问题,2011 年,北京多家医院推出了统一的预约挂号平台,患者可以在线挂号或电话挂号。

_____

_____

5. 当时我父母从中国来看我。一个普通的发烧在美国竟然需要走这么多程序,花那么多钱,这让他们简直难以置信。

_____

_____

VI. Further Readings

1. History and Development of Public Health
2. A Few Thinking about Public Health Development in China
3. Regional Action Plan on Health Promotion in the Sustainable Development Goals: 2018 – 2030

Part II ： Academic Development

I. Translating Medical Texts

Read the following sample abstract and put the underlined part into English.

【摘要】医疗卫生事业是重大的民生工程,医疗卫生体制改革是世界性难题。在中国共产党的领导下,新中国医疗卫生事业取得的成就被世界卫生组织誉为“发展中国家的典范”。医疗卫生事业发展既有经济性因素,也是政党价值观最鲜明的体现。中国共产党以人民为中心的发展宗旨,决定了医疗卫生事业发展的超经济属性。党执政理念的不断进步,推动了医疗卫生事业发展螺旋式上升。进入新时代,要着眼新发展阶段、新发展理念、新发展格局,将医疗卫生事业作为推动构建新发展格局的重要力量;将医疗卫生制度提升到建设现代化国家的基础性制度安排;将全面深化医疗卫生体制改革作为推进健康中国建设的关键内容。①

_____

① 选自《管理世界》2021 年第 11 期,26 – 40 页。作者:费太安。

Translation & Writing Skills: Combine Sentences

English tends to have long and complicated sentences while Chinese tends to have short and simple sentences. It is necessary to combine Chinese simple sentences into English compound or complex sentences. Therefore, it is an important translation skill to combine sentences in translation.

Example 1:
①战士无所畏惧地奋勇向前。②他的脚步很坚定。
Fighters march forward fearlessly, with firm steps.

In this example, The Chinese simple sentence "他的脚步很坚定" is converted into a prepositional phrase "with firm steps" in the translated text to indicate the manner.

Example 2:
①事实并不是这样。②生活并不是一个悲剧。③它是一个"搏斗"。
However, that is not how things are, for life is not a tragedy, but a "struggle".

In this example, there are three simple sentences in the original Chinese text, which have close relationship with one another. In the English version, they are combined into one complex sentence with the conjunction "for" leading an adverbial clause which indicates the reason.

Example 3:
①最后两个字是特别用力的。②大家都不懂"这个"是什么。
He laid special stress on the word "this", but nobody appeared to understand what he meant.

In the above example, the two simple Chinese sentences are combined into one compound English sentence, connected by the coordinating conjunction "but", which shows a transition.

Example 4:
①此外,同一年龄组根据不同性别分为 2 组。②儿童组又根据造血特点将其分为儿童 1 组[48 名,年龄 6(3~7)岁]和儿童 2 组[286 名,年龄 11(8~14)岁]。
Besides, the same age group was divided into two groups according to gender while the children group according to different hematopoietic characteristics were divided into two subgroups: children group 1 [n = 48, 6(3 - 7) years old] and children group 2 [n = 286, 11(8 - 14) years old].

The translation above combined the two short and simple Chinese sentences to form a longer English sentence. Readers of the English version can easily understand on what basis and how the subjects are divided for the research purpose.

II. Writing Medical Papers in English

ABC's of Writing Medical Papers in English
By Todd H Baron

Writing papers can be extremely difficult for those whose first language is not English. The importance of publishing papers in English is based upon several factors: ①English remains the most commonly used language for medical publications (both online and the traditional paper format); ②Most of the higher impact factor journals are published in English; ③Publications in English improve visibility of the author and institution and can be vital to one's academic promotion. Since there are no specific rules about how to publish in English and few references to guide an author on how to publish in English, the following review is based mostly on this author's personal experience in publishing over 300 MEDLINE indexed articles and are what I consider to be the most helpful tips for writing papers in English and for increasing the chances that your manuscript will be published. A helpful web site for information on publications is provided by the ICJME (International Committee of Medical Journal Editors) at http://www.icmje.org/.

Basic Principles

You have only one chance to make a good first impression. When a manuscript is reviewed it has the best chance of acceptance on the initial (and sometimes only) review. While the vast majority of manuscripts are published on their merit, there is subjectivity that can sway the reviewer toward a positive decision. This subjectivity is often based upon how the paper is presented to the reader (in this case, the reviewer) and can be nearly as important as the scientific quality of the manuscript. An analogy is the "presentation" of a meal. While one meal may taste just as good as another, the one with the better presentation is likely to be judged superior. In a manuscript the "presentation" is in the writing style, neatness (correct syntax, lack of misspelled words and typographical errors), and quality of images, tables, and references. Close attention to detail (such as spell checking) can improve the look of the paper and thus its perceived quality.

Select the Correct Journal

There are several considerations when selecting the appropriate journal to submit a manuscript to. This is based not only on the topic, but also on the strength of the manuscript and its appropriateness to the "audience" (type of reader).

High impact factor journals that tend to emphasize basic science or clinical articles are unlikely to accept manuscripts. However, the scientific strength of a manuscript may overcome this obstacle. Procedural papers that are well-designed, well-powered, randomized trials, and those that have broad applicability to clinical care (e. g. procedures that affect the outcome of variceal bleeding) can be published in such journals. Scientific quality of the manuscript can be difficult for an author or authors to address objectively and realistically. However, the greater the scientific quality of the manuscript, the greater the likelihood that it will be accepted in a journal with a high impact factor.

Another consideration in selection of a journal is for the author to select the journal's audience. For example, a predominantly surgical or transplant journal is unlikely to accept a paper that is based on endoscopic or interventional radiologic techniques unless they can integrate them into surgery. Examples include articles about radiologic or endoscopic treatment of post-transplant complications or alternatives to surgery for specific situations (high-risk or non-operative patients).

When selecting the correct journal, you must also assess whether the particular journal has recently published a similar article. If a similar paper has not been recently published, there is generally no effect on the ability to publish the manuscript. However, if a similar article has been recently published, it can either help or hinder the consideration of a manuscript. For example, if the planned manuscript with similar methods shows similar results to the recently published paper, it is less likely to be considered for publication, as it is no longer considered novel. There are three exceptions: ①A manuscript that has results that are in contrast to a recently published study and that show an opposing view creates controversy and diversity (which then increases interest); ② Alternative techniques are used, yet show the same results demonstrating there is more than one method to approach a difficult disorder; and ③Manuscripts where a similar article is submitted simultaneously by another author. In this case, the editor may choose to publish both in the same issue of the journal to create a theme for that issue.

Often, more than one journal could be an appropriate home for an article. Once the author(s) have narrowed their selection to a few journals, it is best to choose the journal with the highest impact factor. Generally, the impact factor is a reflection of the quality and reputation of the journal, and the manuscript will likely generate greater recognition and potentially have a greater influence both on stimulating others to write similar articles and/or influencing patient care. A good overview of the importance, calculation, and flaws of the impact factor is available. The impact factor of a specific journal can be found through ISI Web of Knowledge.

A final consideration when deciding on a journal is whether the author would like to influence one type of readership or another. For example, you may choose to submit a manuscript with an endoscopic technique to influence change among other disciplines or to a more regional journal, which may lead to an increase in practice referrals.

Preparing the Manuscript

Once the author(s) have chosen the journal to which they intend to submit an article, the preparation process begins. The authors should carefully review the "instructions for authors" for the particular journal. Nearly all journals have web sites for online submission. The "instructions for authors" page describes the format for each type of article (original article, case report, review, editorial, etc.) and is available online at the journal home page. Such instructions include how to format the abstract, maximum allowable word counts and images, how to prepare images (i. e. jpeg or tiff), need for a cover letter, and disclosure forms. The author MUST follow these instructions carefully to prevent outright and immediate rejection. Although violation of these rules generally does not mean the manuscript cannot be resubmitted, it will likely result in delays.

The next step is to perform a careful literature search to identify similar papers published in English. This serves several purposes: ① It serves as a guide and demonstrates examples of proper wording used in various sections of the manuscript (for example, the Methods section), which can then be written similarly. It must be emphasized that this is to be used only as a guide. You must but be careful not to copy word-for-word what is written, since this is considered plagiarism; ②It provides ideas for the discussion section; ③It allows generation of a reference list.

How to Manage References

References are an important part of a manuscript in several ways. A manuscript in which the reference list does not contain the most important and pertinent articles is considered incomplete. This relates back to the prior section in performing a complete literature search.

One way to create a complete literature search is to find an article that addresses a similar topic using a medical literature search engine such as PubMed (http://www. ncbi. nlm. nih. gov/pubmed/), a free database accessing primarily the MEDLINE database. Using this site, once an article is identified you can use the "Related Citations" link; this will retrieve all related articles which can be sorted by using the link "Display Settings" at the top. Selecting "Pub Date" will sort the articles chronologically. You can also find reviews by using "Filter Your Results" and then select "Review". A tutorial is also provided which demonstrates other options.

When publishing original articles in which there are many prior publications, the manuscript should only include the most recent or largest sample size publications, although you should be sure to include "landmark" studies that all subsequent papers are based upon despite the date of publication.

You must ensure that the references are correct. This includes correct spelling, title, and names and correct correlation in the text. When mistakes are made in the references it reflects poorly on the quality of the authors' work.

There are two ways to avoid incorrect references. One is to use PubMed, select the desired reference(s) and then select "send to". Then in a drop-down, select "file", a file will open and you can copy and paste the citation(s) into the document. Once the reference(s) is(are) identified they can be stored on the site by creating your own account and "collections" (folders) where they will always be available to use for the same or other manuscripts. To use the reference, click on it and choose the option "send to file", copy the reference and paste it into your document.

The references must be in the format requested by the particular journal. For example, many journals request that all authors be listed when there are six or fewer but when there are more than six authors the first three are cited followed by "et al.". These requirements are present in the instructions for authors as previously mentioned.

When writing the manuscript you should use a reference manager. This allows you to add and delete references and reorder them without having to perform a renumbering process manually. This also avoids errors in the references. Although there are many reference managers available such as EndNote, it is important to realize that Microsoft Word has a "built-in" reference manager and thus can be used by anyone who uses Word (which is the software used almost universally to create documents). Thus, when multiple authors are electronically altering (sharing) the document, they can add or delete references without the need for a separate program.

Writing the Manuscript

There are many ways to approach writing a manuscript. Some authors start at the title page and work down through each section (Introduction, Methods, Results, Discussion, Conclusions). Others write an abstract first and expand the document for each section. This may be the easiest and most practical way to begin, especially if an abstract was prepared for presentation at a scientific meeting. However, there is no exact order that must be followed and some authors start with the Methods and Results sections and move to other sections later.

Some general style points are worth noting. You should avoid writing excessively long Introduction and Discussion sections. Indeed some journals now have word or space limits to the Introduction section. In any case, longer (more words) does not equate to better.

The Introduction should do just that: lay the groundwork for the paper. The most important key points should be mentioned with references that lead up to the purpose of writing the paper.

Methods should be written as clearly as possible and in as few sentences as possible. If a method used is similar or identical to one described in a prior publication you can say something like "Pseudocyst drainage was performed as previously described" (with reference). Then say, "Briefly, using a 20 Gauge needle (Model type, Manufacturer, Company location) was passed through a standard duodenoscope (Model type, Manufacturer, Company location) and was used to puncture the area of endoscopically visible extrinsic compression in the stomach or duodenum". You should avoid editorializing in the Methods and Results sections.

The Discussion section should address the most important points you want to make in the manuscript. It needs to be coherent and you should not feel obliged to fill as much space as possible. You should only write what needs to be written to make the points and not to just "fill space". The Discussion section should begin with an introductory basic overarching statement that summarizes what is known about the topic, and what led to the performance of the study. Each subsequent paragraph should contain a single, main point. There should be a transition sentence to the next paragraph, either at the end of the previous paragraph or as the first sentence in the next paragraph. For papers with original data, you must help the reader understand what makes the manuscript unique or different, or confirm what has previously been published.

During the writing process the "track changes" feature of Word should be used when sharing the document between authors. This makes it easier to see changes made by other authors so that everyone is "on the same page". It also allows you to identify which author made these changes and the exact time and date.

Unit 2

Real-World Evidence

📖 **Lead-in** Real-World Data and Real-World Evidence

Task 1 *Watch the video and answer the following questions, and then exchange your answers with your classmates.*

1. Explain "real-world data" and "real-world evidence" in your own words.

_____

_____

2. What is the relationship between "real-world data" and "real-world evidence"?

_____

_____

Task 2 *Watch the video again and fill the following gaps. Make sure the word(s) you fill in is(are) both grammatically and semantically acceptable.*

There's a lot of talk about real-world evidence. That's because there's (1) _____ _____ we can capture and access today with advances in (2) _____ that might help provide new insight into (3) _____ and how to diagnose and treat them.

The FDA has long used it to monitor (4) _____ after drugs have been approved.

The sources of real-world data include things like (5) _____, claims and billing activities, product and disease registries, (6) _____, and data gathered from other sources that can inform on (7) _____ , such as mobile health devices.

Patients are motivated to (8) _____ this data，but patient organizations often lack the (9) _____ needed to build robust data sets that can meet the demands of regulators.

Part I   Intensive Reading

Real-World Evidence：Time for a Reality Check
By John W. Sweetenham

1   The emergence of big data，AI，predictive analytics，and advanced bioinformatics platforms is transforming our understanding of cancer，our approaches to developing new treatments，and our thinking about cancer care delivery and the true value and benefit of new interventions to patients and their caregivers. Realization of the power of these new tools is growing and large data sets，with their associated analytics，have entered the mainstream of cancer research and cancer care. In the last few years，we have started to witness the transition of large data sets from a resource to mine for generation of hypotheses，to a data source which can be used as reliable information to test hypotheses and answer challenging questions，often based on the massive volume of data available.

2   A very tangible example of this is the growing willingness of the U.S. Food and Drug Administration（FDA）to approve new cancer treatments based partly on the use of what has now become known as "real-world data"（RWD）. In fact，the FDA recently issued guidance to industry for the submission of documents using RWD and RWE （"real-world evidence"）for drugs and biologics. The document defines RWD as data relating to patient health status and/or delivery of health care that are routinely collected from a variety of sources including electronic health records（EHRs），medical claims and billing data，product and disease registries，patient-generated data（such as patient-reported outcomes）and mobile devices such as wearables. It defines RWE as the clinical evidence derived from the analysis of RWD.

3   Acknowledgment of the potential contribution RWD can make to our understanding and decision making has been driven by many factors，not least being the challenge of conducting relevant and impactful clinical trials of new therapeutics. The observation that patients recruited to cancer clinical trials are not representative of the general population of patients with cancer is well documented, and not surprising given that only 2% to 3% of all patients with cancer in the US enter onto a study. The reasons for this are multifactorial and complex, including the often stringent eligibility criteria for trials, failure to adequately represent minority populations, inadequate information and education for the public regarding clinical research, and the time constraints of busy clinical practices. As the oncology world attempts to address all of these issues, including relaxing eligibility criteria for trials to make them more representative of the "real world" population, clinical trials still take many months or years from concept to design to completion and the new treatments under evaluation can still sometimes face an uncertain pathway to approval, especially when the benefits observed in some studies can be marginal.

Big Data's Big Problem

4 Recognizing the rapid increase in the number of new cancer therapeutics in the last few years, the FDA has streamlined its approval process—a change which has undoubtedly given our patients access to effective new therapies more quickly than in the past. This has been a positive development but the process is still far from perfect and there are several studies which show that many recently approved drugs do not meet criteria for clinical benefit by widely used value frameworks such as those of ASCO (American Society of Clinical Oncology) and ESMO (European Society of Medical Oncology). The use of RWD and RWE is another strategy to accelerate this process. We should regard this as a positive step—large sets of accurate, validated, and consistently collected data are a powerful research tool.

5 But therein lies a big problem—to be useful, the data need to be accurate, consistently collected, and verifiable to a level comparable with what we expect from a prospective clinical trial. If the data contained within these large sets are anything less, it erodes confidence in what they are telling us. And at the moment, we are seeing an increasing trend toward labeling data sets as "real-world data" when they fall far short of these benchmarks.

6 Why is this concerning? I think there are several reasons, which relate partly to data quality and partly to how we communicate results of studies.

7 A very quick and superficial PubMed search of "cancer" and "real-world data" brings up literally thousands of publications. A quick survey of a few of these shows how quickly the RWD concept has been embraced by the oncology world, and how much the term is being misused. The studies derive their data from multiple sources, including claims data, individual tumor or treatment registries, data platforms directly downloaded from EHRs, cancer registries, or other single-center series of patients not included in prospective trials. We should have major concerns about the quality of these data.

8 It is a real danger that we legitimize flawed data sets by labelling them as "real-world data" when they neither reflect the real world nor can we trust the data. Historically, registry data have been an important source of hypothesis-generating research. I have personally previously published registry data, clearly labelled as such and clearly recognizing the limitations of these data because of the inherent bias in what gets included in a registry and what doesn't. A close look at some recent publications of "real-world data" shows that these are registry data by another name.

9 From a data quality perspective, we need to be very circumspect about the accuracy of claims data and also of data derived from EHRs, many of which do not adequately capture even stage and performance status—two of the most fundamental data elements we would need for our decision making in the clinic. To label studies using these sources as "real world" is suspect and potentially very misleading.

10 Meaning no disrespect to the author, a recent presentation at the American Society of Hematology reported on the outcomes for patients with aggressive B-cell lymphoma who had undergone CAR-T cell therapy but were not eligible for a prospective trial, and were therefore treated with a commercial product according to the FDA indication. The results of this study were reported as real-world experience, yet this is a highly selected, young patient population with good performance status, which bears no resemblance to the real world of this disease, for which the median age at presentation is around 70 years, performance status is frequently poor, and there is a high incidence of comorbidity. The conclusions of this study are still important, but the results need to be reported in the appropriate context.

Resisting the Hype of RWD

11 This may seem overly critical, but it really matters. There is an extensive literature on the use of spin and the choice of language in reporting the results of studies, demonstrating that nuances in language can often imply a more positive or significant outcome than the study actually shows. As the term "real-world data" becomes socialized in the oncology world, we need to be careful that we do not allow the same thing to happen.

12 Without doubt, there are highly reliable big data sets, derived from multiple centers, abstracted according to consistent validated protocols with robust quality assurance and verification strategies. These sets are a valuable resource with great potential for research and care delivery and their value is already being recognized by many research institutions, health systems, and regulatory bodies. These merit the label of RWD. The term should be restricted to platforms like these. Otherwise, we run the risk that incomplete or inaccurate data derived from inherently biased, or poorly characterized patient populations gain a new respectability as real-world data.

13 Since the concepts of RWD and RWE are now firmly embedded in the oncology vocabulary, it's time to make sure they are clearly defined and that, in our scientific journals and at our major meetings, we limit the use of these terms to studies where they are truly merited.

Words and Expressions

predictive /prɪˈdɪktɪv/ *adj*.	be concerned with determining what will happen in the future
massive /ˈmæsɪv/ *adj*.	very large in size, quantity, or extent
routinely /ruːˈtiːnli/ *adv*.	something is done as a normal part of a job or process
potential /pəˈtenʃl/ *adj*.	existing in possibility
stringent /ˈstrɪndʒənt/ *adj*.	of laws, rules, or conditions which are very severe or are strictly controlled
eligibility /ˌelɪdʒəˈbɪlɪti/ *n*.	the quality or state of being eligible
verification /ˌverɪfɪˈkeɪʃən/ *n*.	evidence that provides proof of an assertion, theory, etc.
streamline /ˈstriːmlaɪn/ *v*.	to make an organization or process more efficient by removing unnecessary parts of it
validate /ˈvælɪdeɪt/ *v*.	to prove or confirm that a claim or statement is true or correct
bias /ˈbaɪəs/ *n*.	a tendency to prefer one person or thing to another
benchmark /ˈbentʃmɑːk/ *n*.	a standard by which something can be measured or judged
legitimize /lɪˈdʒɪtəmaɪz/ *v*.	to give legal force or status to; make lawful
circumspect /ˈsɜːkəmspekt/ *adj*.	cautious in what you do and say and do not take risks
comorbidity /ˌkəʊmɔːˈbɪdɪti/ *n*.	the occurrence of more than one illness or condition at the same time
robust /rəʊˈbʌst/ *adj*.	very strong or healthy

I. Reading Comprehension

Choose the best answer to each of the following questions.

1. According to the passage，RWE is defined as _____.

   A. the theoretical evidence derived from analysis of EHR

   B. the clinical evidence derived from the analysis of RWD

   C. the clinical trials derived from the analysis of RWD

   D. the ideal trials derived from the analysis of EHR

2. The two fundamental elements that can help clinicians make clinical decisions are _____.

   A. stage and performance status

   B. quality assurance and verification

   C. electronic health records and claim records

   D. clinical trials and stringent eligibility criteria

3. Why did the author mention the presentation at the American Society of Hematology?

   A. To report the outcomes for patients with aggressive B-cell lymphoma who had undergone CAR-T cell therapy.

   B. To show the significance of the presentation.

   C. To denounce the use of commercial product in treating patients with aggressive B-cell lymphoma.

   D. To illustrate the point that using flawed data sets as RWD can be misleading.

4. What does "the term 'real-world data' becomes socialized" mean in Paragraph 11?

   A. The term "real-world data" is generally known by all members of the society.

   B. The term "real-world data" is widely used in oncology world.

   C. The term "real-world data" is negatively affected by social activities.

   D. The term "real-world data" is well accepted by the general public.

5. Which of the following is NOT the author's opinion towards RWD and RWE?

   A. Registry data are not necessarily RWD.

   B. Resisting the hype of RWD is of great significance.

   C. The FDA should not use RWD to approve new cancer treatments.

   D. The medical community should remain cautious in labeling data as RWD.

II. Vocabulary

Task 1 *Fill in the blanks of the following sentences with the words or expressions given in the box below. Change the forms where necessary.*

merit	comorbidity	nuance	undergo	tangible
circumspect	embrace	concern	embed	define
bias	potential	validity	intervention	eligible

1. Cultural _____ play a role in the use and acceptance of communications technologies in Asia.

2. All sorts of safety _____ can be reported in an unbalanced manner.

3. She suddenly let all the tears in her eyes trickle out, and she _____ him closely.

4. With a growing population of women participating in sports, sex-based differences in vulnerability to brain injury _____ further study.

5. People are more _____ about claiming that new technologies will revolutionize the world.

6. They propose genetic screening for newborns to _____ benefit both the child and the rest of the family.

7. It's a visible, _____ side effect of matter changing form — it's one part of a chemical reaction.

8. Many randomized clinical trials exclude patients who have multiple _____ to ensure the internal validity of the findings.

9. However, the patient and his family members gave up further ablation procedure or surgical _____ after cautious consideration of the potential benefits and risks.

10. The European Working Relative Effectiveness Working Group _____ real-world data as a measure in understanding health-care data collected under real-life practice circumstances.

11. This report is about the outcomes for patients with a certain lymphoma who had _____ CAR-T cell therapy.

12. These _____ criteria ensure that a homogeneous and representative sample is collected.

13. In this study, the author mentioned immortal time _____, which means that, for patients to have been prescribed SGLT-2 inhibitors, they would first have had to take glucose-lowering drugs, and then an SGLT-2 inhibitor was added.

14. Information from both RCTs and real-world analyses is important to confirm the _____ of safety and efficacy data for new agents.

15. The collagen fibers are firmly _____ in the subchondral bone, giving stability to the cartilage.

Task 2 *Under each of the following boxes there are several groups of sentences. In each group a common word or expression is missing. Find it out from the corresponding box according to the meaning and structure of the sentences. The forms of the words and expressions may vary in the sentences.*

robust   comorbidity   eligibility   multifactorial

Group 1

1. _____ criteria for enrollment included a first diagnosis of breast cancer, women who had not undergone biopsy of axillary lymph nodes before the initial CT examination and women who were not pregnant and had no general contraindication for CT imaging.

2. He was quizzed about his age, medical history and _____ for medicaid.

3. Two researchers(ML and JM) independently assessed the _____ of the literature according to the aforementioned inclusion criteria.

Answer: _____

Group 2

1. This chart illustrates the incidence density rate and HR of CHD stratified by sex, age, and _____ between patients with and without hemorrhoids.

2. Interestingly, several NSP genes have previously been implicated in schizophrenia, a neuro-developmental disorder with high _____ to smoking.

3. Charlson _____ index (CCl) scores were used to determine overall systemic health.

Answer: _____

Group 3

1. Some studies suggested the existence of a _____ association between NT-pro BNP levels, as a diagnostic and prognostic marker of heart failure and sRAGE.

2. However, there was strong and _____ evidence that prenatal mood disturbance, using the average of the two prenatal assessments, predicted total sleep problems at both 18 and 30 months of age independent of postnatal mood and the obstetric and psychosocial covariates.

3. In comparing baseline CPSI scores, the nonparametric Wilcoxon rank sum test was used for comparison between groups, since it is _____ with respect to departures from the assumption of normality required by the usual t-test.

Answer: _____

Group 4

1. It is important to recognize that fracture risk is _____. The likelihood of a fracture depends on bone strength as well as the forces applied.

2. Increase in oxidative stress and lipid oxidation caused by infection periodontitis is a _____ disease, and the genetic background of patients as well as the presence of pathogenic bacteria and the immune mechanisms are thus important elements.

3. It is now becoming increasingly likely that the cause of neurodegeneration in PD is _____ in terms of both etiology and pathogenesis. Genetic factors are now known to cause PD in small numbers of patients with a familial form of the disorder.

Answer: _____

| verification | retrospective | aggressive | stringent |

Group 5

1. His _____ study included 8 patients with PCa consecutively treated with CK system.

2. We concurrently investigated whether a similar association could be found in prepubertal children through a _____ study, briefly summarized later.

3. In this _____ cohort study with historical controls, median survival was significantly longer for patients who received split-dose SRS compared to single-dose SRS (30 vs. 16weeks; $p = 0.015$).

Answer: _____

Group 6

1. Meticulous design and _____ testing of cancer-targeted gene therapy in preclinical settings should facilitate a clear path for future applications in clinics.

2. Equal RNA loading was confirmed by hybridization with a GAPDH cDNA probe. All washes were performed under _____ conditions, and transcripts were visualized by autoradiography.

3. It is generally believed that tolerance to self of CD4 T cells is more _____ than for B cells, due to deletion of autoreactive T cells during their development in the thymus (negative selection) and the action of natural regulatory T cells (nTreg).

Answer: _____

Group 7

1. Online megavoltage (MN) imaging was the main mode of prostate IGRT (Image

Guided Radiation Therapy）, with 50% of centers using this _____ technique.

2. The high proportion of 66% of UK centers using CBCT _____ in this survey indicates an improvement in IGRT equipment compared with the 2010 data from the ESTRO-HERO project.

3. In this study, we only focused on dose _____ of the bladder and the rectum for those treated patients. Our results suggest that the current patient instruction with only drink a glass of water is not sufficient to ensure the bladder filing in a busy center.

Answer：_____

Group 8

1. In summary, we report CDH1 alteration as the pathognomonic feature of plasmacytoid variant bladder cancer, a disease subtype with an _____ clinical behavior and poor prognosis.

2. First described in 1989, this is an _____ form of NHL which is universally associated with HHV8.

3. Cancer cells that develop the ability to interfere with those pathways subsequently develop resistance to primary cancer therapies; often, this leads to drug-resistant, more _____ tumors with worse clinical outcomes.

Answer：_____

III. Cloze

Fill in each of the following blanks with the most appropriate word from each of the four choices given.

Real-World Evidence: Experience from China

In China, the concept of real-world evidence arose from awareness of the __1__ of traditional clinical trials, and the need for additional evidence to inform healthcare practice and __2__ decisions. As early as 2002, the Chinese Ministry of Labour and Social Security hosted an academic forum on the use of insurance __3__ data for drug formulary decision and pharmacoeconomic __4__. The term "real-world evidence" was not __5__ used until 2010, when researchers from traditional Chinese medicine carried __6__ a real-world study to evaluate traditional Chinese medicine interventions, mainly to __7__ the complexities of such interventions. Since then, the Chinese research community has started to __8__ the concept, and has adopted the same definition as the international research community, although some terms, such as outcomes research and comparative effectiveness research, which share ___9___ concepts, have also sometimes been used. For instance, the Chinese Medical Doctor Association began to ___10___ outcomes of research in 2012, and the use of observational studies to ___11___ the effects of healthcare interventions. In 2016, the Chinese Evidence-based Medicine Centre organized a national workshop on real world evidence to explain the concept and ___12___ methods of real world studies to the Chinese audience. In 2017, the centre hosted a national academic forum ___13___ the use of real-world evidence in healthcare decision making. In fact, efforts to ___14___ real-world evidence started far earlier than the official introduction of the concept. The first registry in China was the Shanghai Tumour Registry, which ___15___ data from children aged under 15 years between 1973 and 1977.

1. A. empathy   B. regimen   C. limitations   D. coexistence
2. A. organization   B. unit   C. workshop   D. policy
3. A. advance   B. claims   C. disturbs   D. movements
4. A. evaluation   B. assurance   C. insurance   D. concerns
5. A. fairly   B. explicitly   C. heterogeneously   D. freely
6. A. away   B. back   C. out   D. off
7. A. dissect   B. held   C. burst   D. accommodate
8. A. enlarge   B. enrich   C. embrace   D. embed
9. A. overlapping   B. demonstrating   C. confirming   D. conjecturing
10. A. reveal   B. prove   C. pump   D. promote
11. A. corrode   B. assess   C. comfort   D. inhibit
12. A. add   B. diminish   C. increase   D. introduce
13. A. on   B. in   C. out   D. off
14. A. imitate   B. generate   C. hold   D. crash
15. A. confronted   B. compared   C. collected   D. contrasted

IV. Discussion and presentation

Answer the following questions on the basis of your reading.

1. Do you agree with the author's analysis in the section "Big Data's Big Problem"? Why or why not?

2. In Paragraph 7, the author mentions that RWD is misused. Can you share a case with your classmates?

3. What do you know about the research development of real-world evidence in China?

V. Translation

Translate the following sentences into English.

1. 真实世界证据可用于研发医疗产品、支持医疗实践和制定政策。

2. 尽管人们越来越关注真实世界证据在医疗监管和报销决策中的潜在价值,但在 RWE 的收集和使用方面还面临操作、技术和方法学的挑战。

3. 一种常见的错误观点认为,传统的随机对照试验不能反映真实世界的情况,而所有的观察性研究都是真实世界的。

4. 真实世界数据是指通过多种渠道获得的数据,这些渠道与患者健康状况或在常规临床实践中提供的医疗保健和医疗行为有关。

5. 在过去几年中,国家药品监督管理局研究了如何将真实世界证据应用于药品和医疗器械的开发。

VI. Further Readings

1. Real-World Evidence—What Does It Really Mean?
2. Should Real-World Evidence Be Incorporated into Regulatory Approvals?
3. Using RWE Research to Extend Clinical Trials in Diabetes: An Example with Implications for the Future

Part II　Academic Development

I. Translating Medical Texts

Read the following sample abstract and put the underlined part into English.

【摘要】传统的随机对照临床试验在长期使用过程中暴露出一些不足,这促使越来越多的研究者将目光投向真实世界证据(RWE)。真实世界数据(RWD)作为真实世界研究(RWS)的重要基础,决定了 RWS 是否能为监管和审评机构提供可靠的 RWE。<u>目前RWD 在使用过程中存在一些问题,表现为数据非结构化和零碎化、可及性差、数据的标准化处理缺乏数据标准、数据收集所依据的研究设计不严谨、未严格把控 RWD 的适用性等。这些问题极大地影响 RWD 的质量。</u>本文针对以上问题,提出加强对医疗机构中的 RWD 的管理、完善 RWD 的共享机制、RWS 过程中应根据数据标准将 RWD 标准化、RWD 的收集应依据严谨的研究设计、明确与 RWD 质量相关人员的职责、严格把控 RWD 的适用性等 6 条建议,以期解决 RWS 中 RWD 存在的质量问题,为提升 RWD 质量提供参考。①

> ### Translation & Writing Skills：Parallelism

Working on the translation of parallel structures from Chinese to English, the translator should pay attention to the parallelism in English sentences. In English grammar, parallelism is the similarity of structure in a pair or series of related words, phrases, or clauses. By convention, items in a series appear in parallel grammatical form：a noun is listed with other nouns, an *-ing* form with other *-ing* forms, and so on.

Parallelism can be realized in one of the following three ways：

- With a coordinating conjunction such as *and*, *but*, *or*, *nor*, *yet*；
- With a pair of correlative conjunctions such as *either...or...*, *not only...but also*；
- With a word introducing a comparison, usually *than* or *as*.

Examples are shown below：

---

① 选自《中国新药杂志》2021 年第 13 期,1160 – 1163 页。作者：李宛亭,乔佳慧,孟令全,连桂玉,黄哲,陈玉文。

Example 1：

主要终点为院内死亡率,次要终点包括二次开胸止血、肺部感染、术后持续肾脏替代治疗、截瘫、心力衰竭、住院时间及住重症监护病房(ICU)时间。

The primary endpoint was in-hospital mortality, and the secondary endpoints included secondary thoracotomy, pneumonia, postoperative continuous renal replacement therapy, paraplegia, heart failure, length of hospital stay and intensive care unit (ICU) stay time. (parallelled noun expressions)

Example 2：

机器人辅助进行髋、膝关节置换手术的优势不仅在于术前可进行三维手术规划,而且手术过程中机械臂能够辅助完美实现术前规划。

Robotic assisted joint arthroplasty can not only provide 3D pre-operative visual planning, but also can assist to fulfill the pre-operation plan perfectly. (not only v. + but also v.)

Example 3：

PD 运动并发症风险分层治疗方案,在提高 PD 患者生活质量、兼顾改善运动症状和延缓运动并发症方面具有良好效果。

The stratification medical treatment might have a positive intervention effect on promoting a better quality of life, improving motor symptoms and delaying motor complications in PD patients. (v-ing + noun expressions)

Example 4：

目前各类数字骨科技术如虚拟现实、导航辅助系统、个性化截骨和机器人辅助手术等在关节外科应用如火如荼。

At present, various digital orthopedic technologies such as virtual reality technology, navigation assistance systems, and patient-specific instrumentation (PSI) and robot-assisted surgery in joint surgery are in full swing. (such as + noun expressions)

II. Writing Medical Papers in English

Writing an Effective Title

By Zahra Bahadoran, Parvin Mirmiran, et al.

Good titles are created with care and craft. Writing a good title needs a back-and-forth process by continuous going back to the text with a sharper focus on what the paper is trying to say. As shown in Figure 1, a stepwise process is suggested to be followed to draft a title.

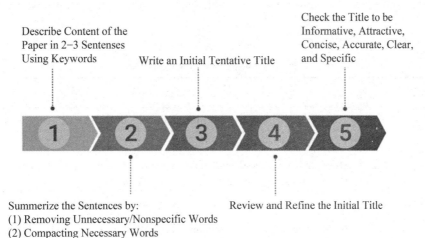

Figure 1   A five-step process of writing a title for a research paper

What the authors need to do in the first step is to consider the manuscript entirely and then try to describe the content of the paper using essential keywords and phrases. Then, they need to make a sentence by the selected keywords and then remove redundant and nonspecific words/adjectives. The keywords used in the title should be the same as that used in the question and answer in the introduction, discussion, and abstract.

The initial title must then be reviewed, refined and finally checked for having features of an effective final title. The title should not be hastily finalized; making a consultation with colleagues to get their opinion and possible suggestions can help improve the title. The authors are highly recommended to adhere to the style of the journal that they are submitting to e. g. word count, other instructions such as acceptable types of title (declarative and interrogative ones are unacceptable by some), use of capital letters, hyphens, colon, etc.

Features of a Suitable Title

In addition to highlighting the subject matter (be informative), the title of the paper should be eye-catching (be attractive). The most important concept should be placed at or near the beginning of the title (where it most readily catches the reader's eye). **Table** 1 describes the features of a good title.

Length of the Title

Although longer titles may provide more information regarding the content, they reduce the interest generated. A short title is easier to understand and can attract a wider readership and increase the influence of the paper. Therefore, the authors are advised to make the title as short as possible without sacrificing accuracy, completeness, specificity, and clarity. High-impact journals usually restrict the length of their papers' titles.

Table 1   Features of a Suitable Title

Features	How to Be
Being informative	Present essential and enough information about the study
	Use study keywords and key terms
	Inform readers about independent variable, dependent variable, observed effects, and study population
Being accurate	Provide the content or state the message as that used within the text
Being specific	Use specific instead of general words or phrases to make the paper more retrievable (e. g. state the type of education instead of stating it alone when the paper is about nurse education)
	Provide important details (e. g. vitamin D and pneumonia vs vitamin D deficiency and risk for severe pneumonia in children under five)
	Do not use unspecific words as much as possible
	Use "and" correctly (e. g. to join two parallel terms instead of joining the independent and the dependent variables)
Being concise	Omit unnecessary words
	Omit "the" at the beginning of the title (not before singular nouns later in the title)
	Do not use unspecific words such as "a study of" "investigation of" or "observation on"
	Do not use phrases like "role of" "effect of", and "treatment of"
	Do not use some adjectives such as "new" "improved" "novel" "validated", and "sensitive"
	Compact necessary words using category terms, adjective instead of noun (e. g. "reduced" instead of "reduction in"), and noun clusters
Being unambiguous (clear)	Do not use noun cluster, abbreviation, and jargon

Try to keep your title shorter than 100 characters (i. e. letters and punctuation marks), including spaces (120 characters are considered the upper limit). As the rule of thumb, 10 – 12 words may be the ideal length of a title.

Word Choice in the Title

In addition to being relevant to the target audience, every word (excluding articles

e. g. *the* , *a* , *an* , and prepositions e. g. *to* , *about* , *on*) used in the title should add significance. Words in the title need to be checked by Medical Subject Headings (MeSH). Using study keywords to formulate a title is highly recommended. Using the most important keywords in the title is essential for appropriate indexing purposes and for retrieval by search engines and available databases. Indexing services (e. g. PubMed) and search engines (e. g. Google) use keywords and terms in the title. Titles should not start with a numeral, or expressions like "a study of" "a contribution to" "investigations on" or "some interesting". "Influence of" does not evoke much curiosity and if possible should be avoided.

Generally, the use of neutral words (e. g. *inquiry* , *analysis* , *evaluation* , *assessment* , etc.), that give no information to the readers, is not recommended. However, in some cases, these words may be necessary to inform the scope, intent, or type of a study. Although the use of catchy phrases or non-specific language is not recommended in academic writing, they can be used within the context of the study.

Adjectives (e. g. *increased*) that modify quantitative words (e. g. *metabolic rate*) are different from those (e. g. *improved*) that modify qualitative words (e. g. *performance*). Some adjectives such as "novel" or "innovative" need to be replaced by more explicit adjectives to explain to the readers what makes the study novel; e. g. "A noninvasive method of predicting pulmonary-capillary wedge pressure" or "An ultrasound method for safe and rapid central venous access". If possible, replace long words with short ones. Try to avoid gerunds (verb forms that end in -*ing*) in the title as the actor is obscured. Avoid using generic terms such as animal, bacteria, or antibiotic as key terms.

Abbreviations confuse readers and usually are not used by indexing services. In some situations, e. g. long or technical terms in scientific writings, the use of abbreviations can be useful. Using abbreviations that appear as word entries in Webster's Collegiate Dictionary, which are better known than their words (e. g. *DNA* , *AIDS* , and *FDA*), or abbreviations for chemicals (e. g. N_2O_5), is acceptable in the title.

Word Order in the Title

Paying attention to syntax (word order) in the title is important because it can influence the reader's interest in the paper. Generally, words at the beginning of the title make the most impact. Put an important word (e. g. independent or dependent variables) first in the title to attract readers. What you want to be emphasized as the primary subject matter, i. e. , the key concept of the paper needs to appear first and near the beginning of the title. Because search engines such as Google, typically show only the first 6 – 7 words of a title, most associated terms should, therefore, appear

---

earlier. Using a subtitle (to state-specific topic) following the main title (to state general topic) is a technique for putting an important word or phrase first in the title; e.g. "Holistic Review: Shaping the Medical Profession One Applicant at a Time" or "Medical School Admissions: Applicant Projections Revisited".

Use of Preposition in the Title

A preposition is a word or a group of words used before a noun, pronoun, or noun phrase to show direction, time, place, location, spatial relationships, or to introduce an object. The correct use of prepositions in the title makes it more clear and helps the reader to understand how the title elements are related to each other. Typical prepositions used in the title are *by* (to indicate how something is done), *for* (referring to a purpose), *from* (referring to the origin of something), *in* (referring to a location), *of* (belonging to or regarding).

Running Title

To identify the articles in a journal, short phrases called running titles (running heads) appear at the top or bottom of every page or every other page. Running titles are short versions of the title and help readers to keep track of the article throughout its printed pages. As running titles mostly cannot be longer than 50 characters (including the spaces), authors are recommended to use standard abbreviations and omit the study design. In hypothesis-testing papers, the running title usually names independent and dependent variables. The form "X and Y", which is unspecific for the title can be used for the running title.

The essence of research is reflected in its title, which acts as a "signpost" for the main topic of the paper. In addition to presenting the message of the paper, the title should evoke interest in reading the paper. Appropriate types of a title (e.g. descriptive, declarative, interrogative) should be selected by the authors and in all cases, the title should be accurate, unambiguous, interesting, concise, precise, unique, and should not be misleading. The title should present the substance of the work in a clear way.

Unit 3

Health Literacy

Lead-in Health Literacy Basics for Health Professionals

Task 1 *Watch the video and answer the following questions, and then exchange your answers with your classmates.*

1. Can you explain what is "health-literacy" in your own words?

_____

_____

2. What might be the benefits of being health-literate patients?

_____

_____

3. What benefits can health-literate partners bring?

_____

_____

Task 2 *Watch the video again and fill the following gaps. Make sure the word(s) you fill in is(are) both grammatically and semantically acceptable.*

Health care providers have a role in building a (1) _____ with patients and delivering messages in a way that patients can understand. This takes very little time during an office visit. **"Ask Me Three"** are three (2) _____ questions including:

    a. What is my main problem?

b. What do I need to do?

c. (3) _____

Health care providers may take the following 7 strategies to help promote health literacy and ensure that patients are informed and proactive with their health care.

—Look for clues. Some behavioral signs and verbal cues can be indicators of low health literacy.

—(4) _____ instead of written words are more effective for patients to understand their health condition.

—Use demonstration.

—Highlight or circle any take-home points.

—Use (5) _____ and convey the most important concepts first. Speak slowly and avoid acronyms and jargon.

—Teach back. Tell Dan that when he leaves here today a friend or family member is going to ask him about his visit. What will he tell them? The best patient-provider relationships are partnerships.

—Encourage patients to self-manage and (6) _____ .

These strategies help promote health literacy and ensure that patients are informed and proactive with their health care.

Part I Intensive Reading

What Is Health Literacy?
By Chenxi Liu, Dan Wang, et al.

1 Health literacy, a term first proposed in the 1970s, generally concerns whether an individual is competent with the complex demands of promoting and maintaining health in the modern society. Over the past two decades, increasing attention has been attached to the concept due to its significant benefits to individual and public health and the sustainability of healthcare systems. It is considered particularly important when non-communicable diseases (NCDs) prevail and their corresponding costs are steadily rising, highlighting the need for people to take more responsibility in managing their own health with more effective use of health services.

2 Inadequate health literacy is associated with difficulties in comprehension of health information, limited knowledge of diseases and lower medication adherence, which contribute to poor health, high risk of mortality, insufficient and ineffective use of healthcare, increased costs, and health disparities. The existing evidence seems to suggest health literacy as one of the most promising and cost-effective approaches to overcome the NCD challenges. Many countries have included health literacy as a key priority in their policies and practices, such as the USA, Canada, Australia, the European Union and China. The WHO recommends health literacy as an instrument for achieving several key targets listed in the Sustainable Development Goals.

❸ Despite the realization of the importance of health literacy to human health and extensive studies into this area over the past few decades, there is still a lack of consensus on "what the concept actually represents", which, as an essential research question, has often been overlooked.

❹ The concept of health literacy seems to be very flexible, which allows anyone to identify nearly whatever one wants as health literacy. Over 250 different definitions exist in the academic literature. The unclear and inconsistent interpretations of health literacy are projected to limit the development of valid and reliable measurements, the accurate evaluation and comparisons of health literacy initiatives, and the synthesis of evidence to support strategies for improving health literacy. Furthermore, the confusion of the concept is likely to produce disjointed and even contradictory findings, jeopardising the development and implementation of trustworthy and effective health literacy-related interventions and policies.

❺ Health literacy was commonly conceptualized as a set of knowledge, a set of skills or a hierarchy of functions. Four studies highlighted knowledge as the core in the concept of health literacy. Schulz and Nakamoto identified health literacy as a set of basic literacy, declarative knowledge, procedural knowledge and judgement skills. Declarative knowledge represents people's understanding of factual information about health, while procedural knowledge represents people's understanding of rules that guide people's reasoned choices and actions. In combination, they enable people to acquire and use information in various contexts and govern the competence of different tasks. Similarly, Leena Paakkari and Olli Paakkari defined health literacy as a set of theoretical knowledge, practical knowledge and critical thinking, corresponding to declarative knowledge, procedural knowledge and judgement skills proposed by Schulz and Nakamoto. In addition, **they** argued that self-awareness and citizenship also form a part of health literacy because they represent one's ability to assess oneself in an informed way and to take responsibility to improve health beyond a personal perspective. Rowlands et al. found that health literacy is reflected in people's ability to acquire, understand and evaluate knowledge for health. Shreffler-Grant et al. specified the knowledge regarding the dosage, effect, safety and availability of medicines as health literacy associated with complementary medicines.

6 Arguably, the Institute of Medicine (IoM) presented one of the most influential models of health literacy. The IoM model contains four underlying constructs: cultural and conceptual knowledge, print health literacy (writing and reading skills), oral health literacy (listening and speaking), and numeracy. It has a strong focus on the required skills for people to obtain, process and apply information for the purpose of medical care. This model has attracted support from many researchers.

7 For example, Baker refined the contents of health-related print literacy and oral literacy in general populations. Yip argued that speaking, reading, writing, listening and numeracy are particularly important for people with limited English proficiency. Squiers et al. added negotiation skills into oral health literacy and relabelled it as communication skills. Navigation skills were also proposed by Squiers et al. as an important element in the eHealth context. Sørensen et al. summarised the literature and presented skills to access, understand, appraise and apply information and knowledge as four core skills of health literacy, which can cover all related works that people need to carry on when dealing with health information to improve and maintain health. Mancuso, Oldfield and Dreher emphasised the importance of comprehension skills.

8 Several studies viewed health literacy as a hierarchy of functions, which requires different levels of social and cognitive skills. Nutbeam first proposed the three-level model: functional health literacy, interactive health literacy and critical health literacy. This model was further clarified and expanded by several researchers. In Nutbeam's prototypical model, functional health literacy refers to "basic skills in reading and writing to enable individuals to function effectively in everyday situations"; interactive health literacy covers "more advanced skills to extract information and derive meaning from different forms of communication, and to apply new information to change circumstances"; critical health literacy requires "the highest-level of skills to critically analyse and use information to exert greater control over life events and situations". Schillinger interpreted functional health literacy as literacy and numeracy. Chinn considered critical health literacy as the function of understanding social determinants of health and engaging in collective actions. Sykes et al. believed that critical health literacy covers advanced personal skills, health knowledge, information skills, effective interactions between service providers and users, informed decision making, and empowerment including political actions.

9 The concept of health literacy has been evolving over the past decade. It started with a doubt about the usefulness of "information and knowledge", simply because a highly knowledgeable person may not be able to materialise the benefits of acquired information/knowledge. As a result, some researchers recommended the addition of self-efficacy as a component of health literacy.

10 The conceptual expansion of health literacy came as a result of empirical enquiries into the meaningfulness of health literacy. Unlike the theoretical analyses at an early stage, these studies present empirical evidence for advocating a change in the concept of health literacy. The ability to maintain health using acquired information and knowledge is the utmost goal of the development of health literacy. This requires one to understand her/his own ability and situation and work in partnerships with others for achieving the best possible outcomes. Evidence from the UK shows that most patients, caregivers and health workers consider health literacy as a "whole system outcome" rather than an attribute of individuals.

11 Pleasant points out that none of the existing definitions of health literacy were generated through a robust and rigorous scientific approach. The widely used original definition of health literacy, based on the individual ability to process and use information for health gains, has failed to find its evidence support from an increasing body of recent empirical studies. We propose a renewed definition of health literacy, incorporating all relevant themes identified from the existing studies. Health literacy is "the ability of an individual to obtain and translate knowledge and information in order to maintain and improve health in a way that is appropriate to the individual and system contexts". This definition highlights the diversity of needs from different individuals and the importance of interactions between individual consumers, healthcare providers and healthcare systems for maintaining health. The whole-system view can help people better understand the role of health literacy and what needs to be done for improving health literacy.

Words and Expressions

prevail /prɪˈveɪl/ v.　　　　to exist or be very common at a particular time or in a particular place

adherence /ədˈhɪərəns/ n.　　the fact of behaving according to a particular rule

disparity /dɪˈspærəti/ n.　　a difference, especially one connected with unfair treatment

sustainable /səˈsteɪnəbl/ adj.　　that can continue or be continued for a long time

initiative /ɪˈnɪʃətɪv/ n.　　a new plan for dealing with a particular problem or for achieving a particular purpose

synthesis /ˈsɪnθəsɪs/ *n.*	the act of combining separate ideas, beliefs, styles, etc.
jeopardize /ˈdʒepədaɪz/ *v.*	to expose to danger or risk
conceptualise /kənˈseptjʊəlaiz/ *v.*	to form a concept of
prototypical /ˌprəʊtəˈtɪpɪkl/ *adj.*	of, relating to, or being a prototype
interpret /ɪnˈtɜːprət/ *v.*	to explain the meaning of (something)
evolve /ɪˈvɒlv/ *v.*	to change or develop slowly often into a better, more complex, or more advanced state
materialise /məˈtɪərɪəlaɪz/ *v.*	to cause to appear in a bodily form
empirical /ɪmˈpɪrɪkl/ *adj.*	based on testing or experience
rigorous /ˈrɪgərəs/ *adj.*	demanding that particular rules, processes, etc. are strictly followed
incorporate /ɪnˈkɔːpəreɪt/ *v.*	to include sth. so that it forms a part of sth.
consensus /kənˈsensəs/ *n.*	an opinion that all members of a group agree with
contradictory /ˌkɒntrəˈdɪktəri/ *adj.*	containing or showing a contradiction

I. Reading Comprehension

Choose the best answer to each of the following questions.

1. Why did many countries include health literacy as a key priority in their health policies and practices?

   A. Because health literacy is already thoroughly studied.

   B. Because health literacy is a promising and cost-effective approach to overcome the NCD challenges.

   C. Because the WHO recommends health literacy as an instrument for achieving several key targets listed in the SDGs.

   D. Because inadequate health literacy is associated with high risk of mortality.

2. Which of the following is NOT a result of the lack of consensus on the definition of health literacy?

   A. A lack of valid and reliable measurements for health literacy.

   B. It's hard to evaluate and compare health literacy initiatives.

   C. It's hard to gather evidence to support strategies for improving health literacy.

   D. The inconsistent interpretations of health literacy makes patients feel upset.

3. Who does the underlined pronoun "they" refer to in Paragraph 5?

   A. Schulz and Nakamoto.   B. Leena Paakkari and Olli Paakkari.

   C. Rowlands et al.   D. Shreffler-Grant et al.

4. Who among all the researchers has essentially different view towards the definition

of health literacy?

A. Schulz and Nakamoto.　　　　B. Yip and Squiers.

C. Pleasant.　　　　　　　　　D. Schillinger.

5. Which of the following is true about health literacy according to the passage?

A. Health literacy is multifaceted.

B. Poor health, high risk of mortality, insufficient and ineffective use of healthcare are directly associated with low health literacy.

C. Realization of the importance of health literacy can lead to consensus on the definition of health literacy.

D. The more knowledgeable one is, the more health literate one will be.

II. Vocabulary

(Task 1) *Fill in the blanks of the following sentences with the words or expressions given in the box below. Change the forms where necessary.*

highlight	empirical	initiative	rigorous	hierarchy
refine	clarify	literacy	priority	contradictory
sustainable	concern	interpret	identify	argue

1. This study aimed to _____ "what health literacy represents" through a systematic review and qualitative synthesis of existing studies across different contexts in relation to this complex concept.

2. The new Silk Road program is a significant international _____ with global support and investment.

3. Health literacy is also recognized as a key component of the European health policy framework Health 2020, which contributes to reduce health inequities, strengthen public health and ensure people-centred health systems that are universal, equitable, _____ and of high quality.

4. MindEd is a portal that provides free e-learning to help adults to _____, understand and support children and young people with mental health issues.

5. The series of contributions focusing on _____ data covers some of the major issues and provides valuable information for further readings.

6. In a community whose _____ is potable water, a health literacy intervention on curbing diabetes and cancer may not be quickly accepted and sustained.

7. Those items would need to undergo _____ testing with diverse audiences.

8. It was an open and frank, not structured discussion, that allowed to enrich and ____

____ the final recommendations without altering their essence.

9. While this has long been a public health _____ in promoting health and preventing disease, it is now an increasing challenge to the wider health care systems as people are living longer with multiple long-term conditions.

10. Kwan et al. (2006) furthermore _____ the importance of engaging and equipping all parties involved in communication and decisions about health, including patients, providers, health educators and lay people.

11. Top-down is when policies and guidance are given from the top levels of leadership, then interventions are implemented by the layers of _____ until they reach down to the individual community members.

12. Little is known about the proportion of children with limited health literacy, or about how children _____ and use health information in their everyday lives.

13. The largest proportion of American adults with limited _____ are native-born Caucasian speakers of English.

14. One could also _____ that the diversity of approaches reflects a continual lack of consensus on just what exactly health literacy is, what it means and how it functions—which also seems to be true.

15. Two additional studies on the association of eHL levels and preventive health behaviours produced _____ evidence.

Task 2 *Under each of the following boxes there are several groups of sentences. In each sentence a common word or expression is missing. Find it out from the corresponding box according to the meaning and structure of the sentences. The forms of the words and expressions may change in the sentences.*

| disparity   incorporate   prevail   adherence |

Group 1

1. Although the pharmacoeconomic impact of non-adherence has not been widely examined, it is clear that less than full _____ is associated with lower treatment costs but worse health outcomes.

2. The aim of the study was to examine the influence of _____ to a program of exercises on the clinical outcome.

3. NaHS inhibited leukocyte adhesion in mesenteric venules, and importantly, inhibiting CSE enhanced leukocyte _____ and infiltration.

Answer: _____

Group 2

1. Their analysis of health _____ had led to a very similar perspective for achieving health equity in New Zealand.

2. The apparent _____ between levels of HO-1 expression detected by Western blot and the greater increase in HO-1 enzyme activity is well known.

3. Several authors have shown that these disorders are commonly found in clinical practice, although there is some _____ in the prevalence reported in the various published studies.

Answer: _____

Group 3

1. Unlike quantitative methods, qualitative methods _____ a flexibility that enables researchers to be adaptable to the context of the research situation and to respond to the uniqueness of participant contributions

2. The five included studies _____ an additional level of analysis beyond the individual level that led them to be included in this meta-narrative review.

3. There are initiatives that _____ health literacy inside government departments.

Answer: _____

Group 4

1. At the levels of poor fetal growth and insulin resistance that _____ in India, even young children are unable to maintain glucose homeostasis.

2. The most _____ view of HBV's oncogenic role in HCC development is that the viral infection, which spans over decades, induces continuous regeneration of hepatocytes.

3. The patient and their family have their own logic in utilizing healthcare services and these may or may not be in alignment with the _____ logic of healthcare professionals.

Answer: _____

gain	evolve	consensus	exert

Group 5

1. Nevertheless, there is also no _____ among thoracic surgical oncologists or sarcoma specialists as to what disease burden represents an unresectable case.

2. As of 2000, a _____ document published by the Eastern Association of the Surgery of Trauma still recommended that 3-view cervical films (Anterior/Posterior/Lateral/Open mouth) be performed for all level-1 trauma patients with suspected

cervical spine injury。

3. In order to reach a _____ on the optimal technique and considering that most studies include a small number of patients，the authors recommend prospective clinical studies with an independent observer.

Answer：_____

Group 6

1. In this paper，we are aimed at _____ knowledge on the pathways related to several mechanisms used for iron metabolism and virulence in P. salmonis.

2. Cross-sectional studies show that smokers weigh less than age-matched non-smokers，while longitudinal data show that most smokers _____ weight after smoking cessation.

3. Future studies should compare general binocular dysfunctions in populations of all ages in order to _____ a better understanding of their prevalence criteria，special characteristics of the populations，and the study area.

Answer：_____

Group 7

1. As experience grows and ideas _____ further，the term will need to be regularly assessed for its meaning and relevance.

2. Chronic infection with HBV can _____ in liver cirrhosis and hepatocellular carcinoma.

3. Time will show how health literacy will _____ further in policy，research and practice world wide.

Answer：_____

Group 8

1. Oestrogens are known to _____ multiple effects on the development and regulation of the immune system.

2. Various GSK-3 inhibitors _____ neuroprotective effects in a wide array of different neuronal death paradigms.

3. Insulin may _____ a direct influence through estrogen receptors，altering the biologic behavior of steroid hormone target tissues.

Answer：_____

III. **Cloze**

Fill in each of the following blanks with the most appropriate word from each of the four choices given.

In response to surveys that have indicated high rates of poor health literacy in populations, governments and national agencies in countries as diverse as the US, China, Australia and some European nations have developed national strategies and targets to improve health literacy in their populations (Chinese Ministry of Health, 2008; USDHHS, 2010; ACSQHC, 2014). As these policies and other government responses have __1__, increasing attention has been given to interventions to address the challenges posed by __2__ health literacy in populations and to improve health literacy in populations.

Health literacy can be improved through the __3__ of information, effective communication and structured education. It can be regarded as a measurable outcome to health education or patient education. Improvements in health literacy can be __4__ through the measurement of changes to the knowledge and skills that enable __5__ and more autonomous health decision making. Differences in communication methods, media and content will result in different learning outcomes and associated behavioural and health outcomes. In turn, individual responses to information and education will be __6__ by the environment in which they occur.

To date, the majority of research into health literacy has focused on the development of effective __7__ for use in clinical practice. There are __8__ reasons for this in healthcare systems where there is a need for more effective prevention, a commitment to patient-centred care, and greater than ever dependence on patient __9__ of chronic conditions. Research from the European Health Literacy Survey (HLS-EU) has demonstrated that there is a strong social __10__ in the population, with lower levels of health literacy much more common among the socially and economically disadvantaged—indicating that those with __11__ need are generally least able to respond to the demands of the healthcare system.

As indicated earlier, the effects of poor health literacy can be __12__ by improving both the quality of health communications and by improving the sensitivity and practical skills of health professionals to the impact of low literacy on individuals. In addition, increasing attention is being given to __13__ the organisational and administrative complexities faced by patients in using the healthcare system. This is leading to __14__ to patient registration procedures, greater flexibility in making appointments and improved way-finding in hospitals and health clinics.

Practical responses to the challenges of poor health literacy can be __15__ in a range of adaptations to traditional patient and population health education methods in print, broadcast and increasingly in digital and mobile communication, as well as closer attention to improved interpersonal communication between clinicians and their patients.

1. A. increased   B. proposed   C. emerged   D. required
2. A. low   B. patient   C. people's   D. individual
3. A. distribution B. sharing   C. search   D. provision
4. A. obtained   B. demonstrated   C. assessed   D. created
5. A. well-established   B. well-informed
   C. well-reformed   D. well-organized
6. A. moderated   B. monitored   C. marginalized   D. multiplied
7. A. measurements   B. interventions
   C. solutions   D. countermeasures
8. A. complete   B. multiple   C. complicated   D. compelling
9. A. cure   B. treatment   C. self-management   D. self-reliance
10. A. gradient   B. impact   C. distance   D. problem
11. A. proper   B. immediate   C. urgent   D. greatest
12. A. migrated   B. mitigated   C. mounted   D. marked
13. A. correcting   B. intensifying   C. increasing   D. simplifying
14. A. modifications B. rectifications C. standardization   D. ramification
15. A. realized   B. improved   C. observed   D. widened

IV. Discussion and Presentation

Answer the following questions on the basis of your reading.

1. Different definitions cover different aspects of health literacy, so what aspects are mentioned among the definitions in the reading?
2. Do you think health literacy is more of an individual property or a community one?
3. Health literacy is an important indicator in measuring basic national public hygiene and health level. Read more reference materials to find out the current status of health literacy among Chinese population.

V. Translation

Translate the following sentences into English.

1. 《上海宣言》还注意到需要跨部门和跨地区的政治行动,强调良好治理和健康素养在增进健康方面的作用以及市政当局和社区所发挥的关键作用。

_____

2. 关于健康素养的承诺包括制订国家和地方策略以提高公民对健康生活方式的认识,以及通过发挥数字技术的潜力,增强公民对自身健康及健康决定因素的控制。

_____

3. 市长们一致承诺将健康作为所有政策的优先考虑,通过多种平台,包括学校、工作场所、现代技术等促进社区参与增进健康。

_____

4. 解决健康和公平问题需要政治承诺、行动和投资,仅靠卫生部门无法确保人们实现最高健康水平。

_____

5. 健康素养还包括一系列广泛的技能和能力,人们通过这些技能和能力寻找、理解、评估和使用健康信息和概念,做出明智的选择,降低健康风险,提高生活质量。

_____

VI. Further Readings

1. WHO Policy Brief for Health Literacy

2. International Handbook of Health Literacy

3. Adolescent Health Literacy in Beijing and Melbourne

Part II Academic Development

I. Translating Medical Texts

Read the following sample abstract and put the underlined part into English.

【摘要】2013 年我国城乡居民健康素养水平为 9.48%,农村居民为 6.92%,城市居民为 13.80%;东部地区居民健康素养水平为 12.81%,西部地区为 6.93%,中部地区为 7.10%;女性健康素养水平为 9.73%,男性为 9.23%。<u>以知、信、行为导向,城乡居民基本健康知识和理念素养为 20.42%,基本技能素养为 12.47%,健康生活方式与行为素养为 10.62%。以健康问题为导向,城乡居民慢性病防治素养为 11.59%,传染病防治素养为 17.12%,基本医疗素养为 8.30%,安全与急救素养为 43.53%,科学健康观素养为 32.12%,健康信息素养为 18.46%。</u>调查表明,我国城乡居民健康素养总体处于较低水平,存在城乡、地区和人群差异。①

> **Translation & Writing Skills: Statistics and Data in Research Papers**

Research papers are always more interesting and convincing if they contain data or statistics. Some research numbers and results can add a really surprising or interesting twist to your papers. When translating the Chinese sentences with statistics or data into English, simple sentence patterns are preferred.

Example 1:
由于无线电波传播的速度是每秒 186,000 英里,声波是每小时 700 英里,因此广播的声音不仅在同一间播音室可以听到,还能在 13,000 英里以外被接收到。

Because radio waves travel at 186,000 miles per second and sound waves saunter along at 700 miles per hour, a broadcast voice can be heard sooner 13,000 miles away than it can be heard at the back of the room in which it originated.

Example 2:
一支铅笔可画一条长达 35 英里的线,或者书写大概 50,000 个英语单词。

The average lead pencil will draw a line 35 miles long or write approximately 50,000 English words.

---

① 选自《人口研究》2016 年第 2 期,88 - 97 页。作者:姚宏文,石琦,李英华。

Example 3:

治疗组病患护理 7 天、14 天、21 天的 NIHSS 评分分别为(12.46±3.25)分、(8.05±2.44)分和(5.49±1.27)分,均低于一般组病患的(20.59±6.18)分、(17.14±5.74)分和(14.59±4.49)分。

NIHSS scores of patients in the treatment group for 7 days, 14 days and 21 days were (12.46 ± 3.25), (8.05 ± 2.44) and (5.49 ± 1.27) respectively, which were lower than (20.59 ± 6.18), (17.14 ± 5.74) and (14.59 ± 4.49) of the general group.

Example 4:

观察组病患对护理工作的总体满意度为 100.00%,对照组病患对护理工作的总体满意度为 87.50%。

The general satisfaction with nursing work of patients in observation group is 100%, while the compared group is 87.50%.

Tips for Using Statistics/Data

- Data plays an important role as evidence to support your thesis. Your paper should contain a good mixture of evidence from a variety of sources, as well as well-constructed discussion points.
- Be sure that you understand the context of statistics you use.
- If you are planning a paper, you will need to use statistics wisely and sparingly. Dramatic statistics are more impactful and easier for your reader to understand in a verbal delivery.

II. Writing Medical Papers in English

Abstract Writing for a Medical Science Journal Article

Writing a scientific article for journal publication can be a daunting task for young inexperienced authors. Although all sections of a manuscript are important and should be well written, the abstract is usually the first section to be read and its content can either attract or repel a reader. Notwithstanding the emphasis given to good manuscript preparation and guidelines provided by journals, many authors still find it hard to produce manuscripts that are compelling or abstracts that are enticing to readers.

As a brief summary, the abstract is expected to be an exact reflection of the content of the main text. It should not contain any information that is not presented in the main text, nor is it expected to exclude vital findings or shortcomings of the research. The emphasis should be on the novel features of the article, and it should be presented logically along the lines of the sections of the article's main text. This includes context and background, objectives, the setting of the research, work done or materials and methods, findings/results, and conclusions from the results. The following lists the features of a good medical science journal abstract:

1. It is a brief summary of completed or ongoing research article;
2. It includes information on the context or background of the study;
3. It states the rationale for the study;
4. It has clear objectives/project statement;
5. It has a succinct presentation of the work done;
6. It contains clear and logical presentation of findings;
7. Its conclusions are supported by the results;
8. It includes a take-home message or statement of impact;
9. It has been written according to journal guidelines: structured or unstructured, word limit, etc.
10. It has good grammatical writing.

Sections of an Abstract

Context/Background: This section of the abstract answers the questions: Why did you start? What is the article about? Why is it important? This should be stated in one or two sentences. Two examples will illustrate this.

Example 1a: *In north India, vitamin A deficiency (retinol $<0.70 \mu mol/L$) is common in pre-school children and $2-3\%$ die at ages $1.0-6.0$ years.*

Example 1b: *Large health surveys use subjective (self-reported) and objective (biomarkers) measures to assess heath status. However, the linkage or disparity of these measures has not been systematically studied in developing countries.*

These examples used one to two sentences each to summarize the respective purposes and importance of the research.

Objectives: You may use one sentence to summarize the aims or objectives of the article. Some journals do not include background material in their abstracts, so the objectives may be the opening section of the abstract.

Example 2a: *To describe the use of mifepristone in combination with buccal misoprostol in women undergoing an early medical abortion (EMA) in Australia.*

Example 2b: *The purpose of this study was to evaluate the effectiveness of a community-based health promotion program targeting people with hypertension and high cholesterol.*

Methods/Setting/Work Done: In this section, you are expected to provide a concise description of study design & methodology used in the study. Because this section provides a lot of information, it should be generally comparatively longer than the previous two sections. Take a look at one example:

Example 3: *Participants in this cluster-randomised trial were pre-school children in the defined catchment areas of 8338 state-staffed village child-care centres (under-5 population 1 million) in 72 administrative blocks. Groups of four neighbouring blocks (clusters) were cluster-randomly allocated in Oxford, UK, between 6-monthly vitamin A (retinol capsule of 200000 IU retinyl acetate in oil, to be cut and dripped into the child's mouth every 6 months), albendazole (400 mg tablet every 6 months), both, or neither (open control). Analyses of retinol effects are by block (36 vs 36 clusters). The study spanned 5 calendar years, with 11 6-monthly mass-treatment days for all children then aged 6-72 months. Annually, one centre per block was randomly selected and visited by a study team 1-5 months after any trial vitamin Ato sample blood (for retinol assay, technically reliable only after mid-study), to examine eyes, and interview caregivers. Separately, all 8338 centres were visited every 6 months to monitor pre-school deaths (100,000 visits, 25,000 deaths at ages 1.0-6.0 years [the primary outcome]). This trial is registered at ClinicalTrials. gov, NCT00222547.*

One of the pitfalls of this section includes omitting vital information on the methods used in an attempt to reduce word count. Rephrasing sentences could be helpful while words and phrases that do not add to the understanding of the abstract should of course be removed.

Results: This is usually the longest section of the abstract. Occasionally it may be as long as or shorter than the methods section. You should concisely present your findings including real data! An abstract that contains no real data is not complete. However, abstracts should not contain tables and figures. Presented below is a good example:

Example 4: *The participants had a mean age of 63 years, and 63% were men. After a mean follow-up of 3.4 years, the risk of recurrent stroke was not significantly reduced with aspirin and clopidogrel (dual antiplatelet therapy) (125* *strokes; rate, 2.5% per year) as compared with aspirin alone (138 strokes, 2.7% per year) (hazard ratio, 0.92; 95% confidence interval [CI], 0.72 to 1.16); nor was the risk of recurrent ischemic stroke (hazard ratio, 0.82; 95% CI, 0.63 to 1.09) or disabling or fatal stroke (hazard ratio, 1.06; 95% CI, 0.69 to 1.64). The risk of major hemorrhage was almost doubled with dual antiplatelet therapy (105 hemorrhages, 2.1% per year) as compared with aspirin alone (56, 1.1% per year) (hazard ratio, 1.97; 95% CI, 1.41 to 2.71; $P < 0.001$). Among classifiable recurrent ischemic strokes, 71% (133 of 187) were lacunar strokes. All-cause mortality was increased among patients assigned to receive dual antiplatelet therapy (77 deaths in the group receiving aspirin alone vs 113 in the group receiving dual antiplatelet therapy) (hazard ratio, 1.52; 95% CI, 1.14 to 2.04; $P = 0.004$); this difference was not accounted for by fatal hemorrhages (9 in the group receiving dual antiplatelet therapy vs 4 in the group receiving aspirin alone). (SPS3 Investigators, 2012)*

Conclusion: Here you should present a brief interpretation of the results, stating the implications and making recommendations for action. The conclusions should be supported by the results presented. Limitations of the study may be briefly highlighted. One or two sentences will be okay for this section.

Example 5a: *DEVTA contradicts the expectation from other trials that vitamin A supplementation would reduce child mortality by 20-30%, but cannot rule out some more modest effect. Meta-analysis of DEVTA plus eight previous randomised trials of supplementation (in various different populations) yielded a weighted average mortality reduction of 11% (95% CI 5 - 16, p = 0.00015), reliably contradicting the hypothesis of no effect.*

Example 5b: *Macroeconomic shocks, structural adjustment, and trade policy reforms in the 1980s and 1990s might have been responsible for worsening child nutritional status in sub-Saharan Africa. Further progress in the improvement of children's growth and nutrition needs equitable economic growth and investment in pro-poor food and primary care programmes, especially relevant in the context of the global economic crisis.*

Form, Style and Grammar

Though the abstract is usually the last section of the article to be written, it should not be done in a hurry. Attention to detail with respect to language is important. The abstract should preferably be written in the active voice, objectively, and briefly. Abstracts generally capture the interest of readers by using a simple language appropriate for conveying information in the discipline. The author as his own editor should read and proofread his abstract and be satisfied that it is a true summary of the text. Submitting the article and, in this context, the abstract to colleagues to proofread may be helpful. Authors should remember that brevity is important! The authors should refer to the journal's instruction to authors to ensure the abstract is in the right format. Some journals have their abstracts structured, with specified subheadings. Others use unstructured format. Whatever the format recommended by the journal, the concepts presented in this article are applicable.

Coping with Word-Limits

The word limit required for the abstract varies from one journal to another but generally lies between 100 and 400 words. It is recommended that the draft of the abstract be written completely, and then edited to remove unnecessary sentences and words. Sentences could be restructured to clarify their meaning or reduce the word length. This should continue until the required word length is achieved without removing important points of the abstract.

Unit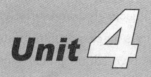

Physician Well-Being

(Task 1) *Watch the video and answer the following questions, and then exchange your answers with your classmates.*

1. Explain what is "physician well-being and burnout" in your own words.

_____

_____

2. Discuss the diagnosis, treatment and prevention of burnout.

_____

_____

(Task 2) *Watch the video again and fill the following gaps. Make sure the word(s) you fill in is(are) both grammatically and semantically acceptable.*

Burnout includes (1) _____

_____

It's caused by (2) _____

_____

It's addressed through (3) _____

_____

To prevent burnout, doctors need (4) _____

_____

Burnout can lead to (5) _____

_____

Part I   Intensive Reading

Medical Student Well-Being: Minimize Burnout and Improve Mental Health Among Medical Students

By Lotte Dyrbye

1 Medical students are at a heightened risk for burnout and depression, and this elevated risk persists into residency. Burnout among medical students has a negative impact on medical student individual well-being and on patient care.

2 Becoming and being a physician is arduous, challenging, and a privilege. Physicians are nearly twice as likely to experience burnout as other US workers, after controlling for work hours and other factors. Burnout is a syndrome of emotional exhaustion, depersonalization (e. g. decreased empathy towards patients), and low sense of personal accomplishment that is primarily attributed to work-related stressors. It is important to understand that the high prevalence of burnout among physicians in practice is not reflective of a problem with admissions or defective personal characteristics. National studies have found that matriculating medical students have better mental health profiles than other similarly aged college graduates who pursue other careers.

3 Once in medical school, however, medical students are more likely to experience burnout and depression than other similarly aged individuals pursuing different careers, and this elevated risk persists into residency. Burnout among medical students predicts developing thoughts of suicide over the course of one year and seriously considering dropping out of medical school. Additionally, burnout among medical students is associated with a 20% increased risk of alcohol abuse or dependence. It is also associated with lower performance on standardized assessments, medical errors, and sub-optimal patient care and professionalism. Burnout and depression prevent medical students from reaching their potential and threaten their professional development.

4 Medical students also experience other forms of distress, such as profound levels of stress, poor quality of life, and high degrees of fatigue. In fact, most medical students experience multiple forms of distress simultaneously, and the more forms of distress they experience the higher their risk is for thoughts of suicide and dropping out of medical school.

5 In addition to accreditation standards, there is a moral and ethical imperative for medical schools to address medical student well-being. Medical schools should take steps to reduce the risk of burnout and depression among their students and make an effort to promote a culture of well-being. This module provides a detailed approach to how this can be accomplished.

6 Following are eight steps to minimize burnout and improve mental health among medical students.

Step 1: Recognize Shared Responsibility

7 Student well-being is a shared responsibility of the individual learner, the school, and course and site faculty where students have clinical experiences. Within the constraints of a demanding schedule and multiple, competing priorities, individual medical students have responsibility for self-care, including engaging in healthy activities, eating nutritiously, sleeping adequately, managing their time, spending time with family and friends, and reaching out for help.

8 From a medical school perspective this responsibility includes implementing and evaluating primary and secondary prevention strategies with appropriate investment in well-being related infrastructure and resources, as well as organizational efforts to reduce drivers of distress. Typically, these strategies include having a dedicated individual (or group) charged with overseeing student well-being who is resourced and empowered to make school-level changes, such as the Assistant Dean of Students, Associate Director of Student Affairs, or Director of Student Well-Being.

Step 2: Measure Student Well-Being

9 Medical student well-being should be a routine performance metric for a medical school. Best approaches include using a standardized instrument with national benchmarks to allow for comparison between how medical students are doing locally versus nationally.

Step 3: Optimize the Curriculum

10 The relationship of many curricular elements to well-being have been examined to date, including hours spent in small lectures and clinical experiences, amount of vacation allocated, number and time devoted to testing, and grading. Of these factors only pass-fail grading was independently associated with reduced risk of burnout. Additionally, research has found that among first and second year (pre-clinical) medical students there is no relationship between hours spent in lectures and small groups, hours of clinical experiences, hours and number of exams, weeks of vacation, and any measure of student well-being, including burnout, quality of life, or depressive symptoms.

11 In particular, a pass/fail grading system is key for decreasing burnout, stress, and serious thoughts of dropping out. In a large multi-institutional study of first- and second-year medical students, those NOT in a pass/fail curriculum had nearly double rates of burnout, higher stress levels, and were 60% more likely to consider dropping out. Switching to pass/fail grading during the non-clinical years does not have a detrimental impact on learning as measured by the United States Medical Licensing Examination (USMLE) Step 1 score or clerkship grades.

12 An excessive workload adds enormous stress to medical students and contributes to limited time for self-care. In addition, required attendance and lack of flexible schedules contribute to their sense of lack of control over their daily lives. Clinical experiences involving excessive administrative tasks or work inefficiencies are also likely to contribute.

Step 4: Help Control Medical Student Debt

13 Approximately 76% of medical students graduate with educational debt. A 2018 analysis from AAMC reported that the median educational debt for medical students graduating in 2017 was $192 000. Educational debt can have a significant impact on a student's overall well-being. In fact, medical school debt is an independent predictor of burnout and increases medical students' risk of alcohol dependence and abuse. In addition, a multi-institutional longitudinal study of 1,701 medical students found that students who worked for income were significantly less likely to recover from burnout over the course of one year than students who were not employed.

Step 5: Optimize the Learning Environment and Cultivate Community

14 Medical students expect to and desire to work hard. It is typically not work hours or clinical workload that lead to burnout, but rather a poor learning environment. This may include inadequate support from faculty, lack of supervision from residents, cynical residents, lack of variety of medical problems seen, and harassment/mistreatment. Therefore, it is essential that students can learn in an organized and supportive environment that promotes their personal and professional development.

Step 6: Promote Self-Care and Resiliency

15 Providing resources to promote self-care and resiliency should be part of every medical school's strategy to promote student well-being. Unfortunately, students have limited time for self-care and this creates a new tension for them as they become role models for patients. Students should be educated to strive for healthy self-improvement and to avoid the self-destructive and exhausting road of perfectionism.

16 Other common experiences include feeling of inadequacy and feeling like an imposter. Dealing with such feelings by having faculty talk about their own experience tends to be helpful. Many schools are trying to emphasize the need for self-care by providing personal days during the clerkship year.

Step 7: Provide Adequate Services for Those Already Affected by Burnout or Distress

17 Despite these prevention efforts, approximately half of medical students experience symptoms of burnout and nearly a third have symptoms of depression. Therefore, medical schools need to take proactive steps to identify students in need of individualized services and provide barrier-free access to mental health care. The Liaison Committee on Medical Education (LCME) has also assessed the need for addressing medical student mental health and has issued specific requirements on standards for accreditation to medical schools.

18 For example, LCME standards state that diagnostic, preventive, and therapeutic health services must be accessible to medical school students near the site of their required educational experiences, which may include classroom facilities, rotation sites, etc. Policies should be in place that allow students to be excused to seek necessary health care.

Step 8: Fund Organizational Science Around Well-Being

19 Research to date has primarily studied the prevalence and factors associated with medical student well-being. Few intervention studies have been conducted, and most of these have focused on individual strategies rather than organizational/medical school level interventions. Although each medical student has a responsibility to engage in self-care, it is system-level factors that are the greatest contributors to medical student distress. Solutions are needed, and for well-designed studies to occur, local investment in novel interventions focused on how to best promote individual healthy choices and improve the learning environment are needed. Vanguard institutions should leverage their faculty to develop evidence-based strategies that other organizations/medical schools can implement. The creation of new knowledge on how best to reduce medical student burnout and enhance their well-being and professional competency development can be achieved through organizational science. Investment is critical to change and to the short and long-term health of medical students.

Words and Expressions

imperative /ɪmˈperətɪv/ *n.*　(formal) a thing that is very important and needs immediate attention or action

accreditation /əˌkredɪˈteɪʃn/ *n.*　official approval given by an organization stating that sb./sth. has achieved a required standard

burnout /ˈbɜːnaʊt/ *n.*　the state of being extremely tired or ill, either physically or mentally, because you have worked too hard

proactive /ˌprəʊˈæktɪv/ *adj.*　(of a person or policy) controlling a situation by making things happen rather than waiting for things to happen and then reacting to them

detrimental /ˌdetrɪˈmentl/ *adj.*　harmful

vanguard /ˈvænɡɑːd/ *n.*　the leaders of a movement in society, for example in politics, art, industry, etc.

imposter /ɪmˈpɒstə/ *n.*　a person who makes deceitful pretenses

matriculate /məˈtrɪkjuleɪt/ *v.*　(formal) to officially become a student at a university

depersonalization /diːˌpɜːsənəlaɪˈzeɪʃn/ *n.*　a psychopathological syndrome characterized by loss of idetity and feelings of unreality and strangeness about one's own behavior

liaison /liˈeɪzn/ *n.*　a relationship between two organizations or different departments in an organization, involving the exchange of information or ideas

module /ˈmɒdjuːl/ *n.*　a unit that can form part of a course of study, especially at a college or university in Britain

admission /ədˈmɪʃn/ *n.*　the act of accepting sb. into an institution, organization, etc.; the right to enter a place or to join an institution or organization

prevalent /ˈprevələnt/ *adj.*　that exists or is very common at a particular time or in a particular place

syndrome /ˈsɪndrəʊm/ *n.*　a set of physical conditions that show you have a particular disease or medical problem

leverage /ˈliːvərɪdʒ/ *v.*　to provide (as a corporation) or supplement (as money) with leverage; also to enhance as

	if by supplying with financial leverage
therapeutic /ˌθerə'pjuːtɪk/ *adj.*	(usually before noun) designed to help treat an illness
arduous /'ɑːdjuəs/ *adj.*	involving a lot of effort and energy, especially over a period of time
longitudinal /ˌlɒŋgɪ'tjuːdɪnl/ *adj.*	concerning the development of sth. over a period of time
diagnostic /ˌdaɪəg'nɒstɪk/ *adj.*	(usually before noun) (technical) connected with identifying sth., especially an illness

I. Reading Comprehension

Choose the best answer to each of the following questions.

1. Which of the following is NOT a negative impact of burnout on medical students?

    A. Developing thoughts of suicide and seriously considering dropping out of medical school.

    B. Being associated with a 20% increased risk of alcohol abuse or dependence.

    C. Being associated with lower performance on standardized assessments.

    D. Reaching their potential and promoting their professional development.

2. According to the passage, the relevant parties are supposed to assume a shared responsibility of promoting medical student well-being EXCEPT _____ .

    A. individual students   B. medical schools

    C. clinical rotation sites   D. governmental agencies

3. Which of the following is NOT an active intervention to minimize burnout?

    A. Evaluating student well-being.

    B. Employing coping strategies of avoidance and denial.

    C. Controlling medical student debt.

    D. Providing resources to promote self-care and resiliency.

4. Which factor was independently associated with reduced risk of burnout?

    A. Hours spent in small lectures.

    B. The amount of vacation allocated.

    C. Number and time devoted to testing.

    D. Pass-fail grading.

5. To promote medical student well-being and minimize burnout, which aspect needs to be strengthened?

    A. The responsibility of individual medical students.

    B. The responsibility of teaching staff.

C. The prevalence and factors associated with medical student well-being.

D. Organizational/medical school level interventions.

II. Vocabulary

(Task 1) *Fill in the blanks of the following sentences with the words or expressions given in the box below. Change the forms where necessary.*

accreditation	attributed	burnout	depression	detrimental
diagnostic	fatigue	heightened	imperative	infrastructure
leverage	proactive	professionalism	resiliency	well-being

1. The fact that it is nurses who of all the health professionals spend the most time with patients at the bedside is another area of potential stress and _____.

2. Little is known of the drug's long term effects on physical health or emotional _____.

3. Researchers have adapted the approach—originally developed for _____ —to manage panic attacks, addictions, eating disorders, social anxiety, insomnia and obsessive-compulsive disorder.

4. Laboratories had completed 13,393,844 total _____ tests for COVID-19 as of Friday, 9.7% of which have come back positive.

5. Healthy people can harbor Klebsiella to no _____ effect; those with debilitating conditions, like liver disease or severe diabetes, or those recovering from major surgery, are most likely to fall ill.

6. He notes that the two would be interesting to study, to see if any of their similarities can be _____ to their genetic connection.

7. Components in honey can help bees live longer, boost their tolerance of harsh conditions such as intense cold and _____ their ability to fight off infections and heal wounds.

8. Thus, it is _____ that health communication scholars focus their efforts on adolescent patient-physician communication.

9. His personality, his _____ and attitude gave Swedish players a good reputation here.

10. Such a _____ approach to liability also accords with modern views of health and safety provisions in general.

11. The drug's side effects include headache and _____.

12. Individuals who meet application requirements will be eligible to sit for the _____

exam.

13. The purpose of a _____ is to attain professional competence in direct patient care and in practice management beyond entry level.

14. They are used by minorities to block legislation and to gain bargaining _____ with majorities.

15. Combining a national investment in public health _____ with a radical shift in rhetoric and messaging about testing will allow the country to effectively respond to what is required in era two of the pandemic.

(Task 2) *Under each of the following boxes there are several groups of sentences. In each sentence a common word or expression is missing. Find it out from the corresponding box according to the meaning and structure of the sentences. The forms of the words and expressions may change in the sentences.*

contribute	intervention	prevalence	therapeutic

Group 1

1. Ireland currently has the highest _____ of asthma in Europe and it is still on the increase.

2. Dementia _____ is higher among those who are physically disabled.

3. The present study also shows a high _____ of ascites in patients with acute liver failure.

Answer：_____

Group 2

1. The effective identification of patients at risk of sudden death must allow possible _____ intervention.

2. These drugs are recommended for the short term treatment（one to two weeks）of acute constipation and as a purgative before diagnostic and _____ endoscopy.

3. If an antidepressant is indicated，it should be used in a full _____ dose and continued for an appropriate period of time.

Answer：_____

Group 3

1. This condition needs medical _____ both in the form of rapid diagnosis and treatment.

2. Bleeding from gastric varices responds poorly to injection sclerotherapy and often

requires surgical _____ .

3. Some women fear a specific _____ , such as being induced, having an emergency cesarean section or going through a forceps delivery.

Answer: _____

Group 4

1. In the absence of such data, local epidemiology and susceptibility patterns may _____ to the empiric selection of therapy.

2. NSAID enteropathy and its complications _____ significantly to the overall morbidity of patients receiving these drugs.

3. The authors concluded that migraine was the most likely neurologic cause of TGA in younger patients, and personality deviation and stress was a _____ factor in women.

Answer: _____

| associated | appropriate | significant | treatment |

Group 5

1. There were no _____ differences between both groups in death, transfusion requirements, and days needed in hospital.

2. Analysis of the data collected in South Wales revealed that there was no statistically _____ difference in the prevalence of dementia or depression across the social class groups.

3. Defining rigorously what constitutes a clinically _____ depressive illness is problematic, regardless of the age range under consideration.

Answer: _____

Group 6

1. Considerable degeneration of the endometriosis occurs after two months of medical _____ , and symptoms should therefore diminish.

2. She is receiving _____ for the weight-loss disorder anorexia nervosa at Rampton top security hospital.

3. The emphasis is on diagnosis and _____ by medical or surgical means and on the measures available for the prevention and control of disease.

Answer: _____

Group 7

1. Oxford is a national centre for the treatment of problems _____ with childbirth, and research in Oxford has made a major contribution to the treatment of these problems.

2. Because HPV-16 DNA is known to activate cellular oncogene and is closely _____ with malignant transformation, these findings suggest that an association of HPV-16 DNA with the multi-step development of colorectal cancers may exist.

3. Dental disease is _____ with an increased risk of coronary heart disease, particularly in young men.

Answer: _____

Group 8

1. For this reason, it's almost always _____ to begin a patient's treatment by correcting any digestive complaints or irregularities.

2. During pregnancy women are advised to consult their doctor about _____ drinking levels.

3. If the patient happens to be older, but is otherwise in good health besides its tumor problem, it is entirely _____ to offer treatment.

Answer: _____

III. Cloze

Fill in each of the following blanks with the most appropriate word from the given choices.

Physician well-being has been studied extensively, __1__ that being a physician is associated with higher levels of stress which can lead to problems both personally and professionally. Some of this stress can be managed on an individual level; however, there are also organizational __2__ that can be helpful.

On an individual level, medical students that had personality characteristics of empathy and self-criticism were more likely to experience __3__ effects on future mental health. In addition to personality types that might predispose to future problems, __4__ coping strategies of avoidance and denial were found to be especially poor outcomes in mental health. Stress begins early in medical training, and __5__ of burnout have been documented in medical students with nearly one half of third-year students reporting burnout and a __6__ between burnout and suicidal ideation in medical students.

On a job level, having high demands or being overloaded is associated with stress. Hours of sleep were __7__ related to depression in one study. Main stressors were relationships with senior doctors, making mistakes, conflict of career with personal life, and litigation fears. For those physicians that were general __8__ and not hospital doctors, dealing with patients was also found to be a __9__. A sense of loss of control and/or loss of meaning may well be __10__ to stress and burnout. Physicians find "being present" with patients correlates strongly with finding meaning in their work. Programs offering __11__ training for primary care physicians in mindfulness have been associated with short term and __12__ improvements in well-being and attitudes associated with patient centered care.

In the Firth study which was __13__ in the UK, smaller organizations had better mental health outcomes with more cooperation, better communication, more performance monitoring, a stronger emphasis on training and allowing staff __14__ discretion over work. Also, hospitals which were found to have good reputations as places to work had lower staff burnout and better patient outcomes than those without the good reputations.

Physician well-being is one of the __15__ of professionalism. Joint Commission on Accreditation of Health Care Organization requires all hospital medical staff to have physician wellness committees or to work with already established physician health programs in the state.

1. A. considered   B. considering   C. providing   D. provided
2. A. commitment   B. involvement   C. interventions   D. participation
3. A. hostile   B. adverse   C. favorable   D. positive
4. A. adopting   B. employing   C. involving   D. choosing
5. A. phenomenon   B. evidence   C. sign   D. symptoms
6. A. distinction   B. correlation   C. similarity   D. connection
7. A. dramatically   B. considerably   C. significantly   D. enormously
8. A. practitioners   B. practice   C. practise   D. practical
9. A. strain   B. tension   C. stressor   D. stress
10. A. related   B. connected   C. associated   D. correlated
11. A. rigorous   B. detailed   C. systematic   D. extensive
12. A. maintained   B. perpetual   C. constant   D. sustained
13. A. undertook   B. organized   C. conducted   D. operated
14. A. more   B. greater   C. better   D. further
15. A. foundations   B. fundamentals   C. principles   D. framework

IV. Discussion and Presentation

Answer the following questions on the basis of your reading.

1. Describe the drivers and importance of medical student well-being.
2. What can be done to optimize the learning environment?
3. How can students recognize the need for self-care?

4. What can students do on an individual level?

V. Translation

Translate the following sentences into English.

1. 这对我们卫生系统的可持续发展和患者的安全构成了重大威胁,当前亟需系统解决职业倦怠的方案。

2. 职业倦怠是一种以高度情绪耗竭、人格解体(即愤世嫉俗)和工作中个人成就感低下为特征的综合征。

3. 组织机构需要全面彻底地了解临床医生职业倦怠的根本原因,才能实施切实有效的解决方案。

4. 临床医生的职业倦怠影响医护团队的所有成员,并对医疗保健系统的效率和有效性产生重大影响。

5. 任何单一的干预措施都不可能有效地解决工作倦怠问题,而解决工作环境问题的多维方法可能最为成功。

VI. Further Readings

1. Prevalence of Burnout in Medical Students in China

2. The Effects of Work-Hour Limitations on Resident Well-Being, Patient Care, and Education in an Internal Medicine Residency Program

3. Patient Safety, Resident Well-Being and Continuity of Care with Different Resident Duty Schedules in the Intensive Care Unit: A Randomized Trial

Part II   Academic Development

I. Translating Medical Texts

Read the following sample abstract and put the underlined part into English.

【摘要】目的：调查临床实习压力对医学生心理健康的影响，为开展实习期医学生心理健康工作提供相关依据和支持。**方法**：采用 Beck-Srivastava 压力量表(BSSI)对 586 名处于临床实习期间医学生面临的压力源及压力强度情况进行初步检测，进一步结合症状自评量表(SCL-90)状态—特质焦虑问卷(STAI)对其心理健康状况进行综合调查。**结果**：①临床实习期间，医学生的压力主要集中在学习压力、经济压力、临床实践和人际关系 4 个方面，其检出率普遍超过 60%，且 BSSI 单因子得分均在 3 分以上。男生在学习压力及经济压力 2 个因子得分高于女生，在临床实践及人际关系 2 个因子得分低于女生，但差异均无统计学意义($P>0.05$)；②临床实习期间医学生在 SCL-90 的 9 个因子得分均超过国内常模，且在人际关系、抑郁、焦虑及恐怖 4 个因子得分差异有统计学意义($t=8.5011, 5.0781, 27.5146, 3.4907; p<0.05$)。男生在 SCL-90 的敌对性、偏执及精神病性 3 个因子得分高于女生，但差异均无统计学意义($P>0.05$)；女生在 SCL-90 的躯体化、强迫、人际关系、抑郁、焦虑和恐怖 6 个因子得分高于男生，且在抑郁和焦虑 2 个因子得分差异有统计学意义($t=-4.2678, -3.7579; p<0.05$)；③临床实习期间医学生在 STAI 的状态焦虑(S-AI)的得分高于标准常模，且差异有统计学意义($t=8.3293, p<0.05$)，在 STAI 的特质焦虑(T-AI)的得分低于标准常模，但差异无统计学意义($P>0.05$)；女生在 S-AI 及 T-AI 得分均高于男生，但差异均无统计学意义($t=-0.5390, -1.4026, P>0.05$)。**结论**：临床实习会对医学生造成较大的压力，进而导致一定的心理健康问题，尤其是会诱发较为严重的焦虑情绪。[①]

> **Translation & Writing Skills：Discourse Markers**

Some words and phrases help to develop ideas and relate them to one another. These kinds of words and phrases are often called discourse markers. Note that most of these discourse markers are formal and used when speaking in a formal context or when presenting complicated information in writing or translating.

1. with regard to/regarding/as regards/as far as...is concerned/as for

These expressions focus attention on what follows in the sentence. This is done by announcing the subject in advance. These expressions are often used to indicate a change of subject during conversations.

---

① 选自《中国健康心理学杂志》2017 年第 4 期，595-598 页。作者：李明，苏伟，周婷，梅瑞华，张秋梅，程刚。

Examples:

- Data *with regard to* the technical quality and appropriateness of clinical care were not available in the electronic system, which limits the evaluation of the effects of medical care factors on patient outcomes.
- There is a case for argument *regarding* the follow-up or surgical resection of mediastinal cysts.
- Furthermore, there were no cohort studies, *as far as* we reviewed, which showed an either significantly positive or negative association of DM with ovarian cancer.
- *As for* the bladder, only a few studies found dose-volume relationships associated with the risk of GU toxicity.

2. on the other hand/while/whereas

These expressions present two ideas which contrast but do not contradict each other. "While" and "whereas" can be used as subordinating conjunctions to introduce contrasting information. "On the other hand" should be used as an introductory phrase of a new sentence connecting information.

Examples:

- The active stage of the disease was found in 22 patients *while* 31 patients were in remission.
- Pain on movement and on deep tissue palpation, *on the other hand*, is probably due to the mechanosensitivity of sites of ectopic electrogenesis.
- It should be taken into account that in some patients risk factors were corrected medically or through lifestyle adaptations, *whereas* in other patients risk factors were not sufficiently corrected.

3. however/nonetheless/nevertheless

All these words are used to begin a new sentence which contrasts two ideas. These words are often used to show that something is true despite not being a good idea.

Examples:

- Smoking is proved to be dangerous to the health. *Nonetheless*, 40% of the population smokes.
- In contrast to the SPR analysis, *however*, these results suggest a different secondary preference of the aPI binding domain from both IQGAP1 and -2.
- Given that seizures do not invariably cause cardiopulmonary arrest, the present case *nevertheless* raises the possibility that primary seizures can play a causative role in sudden infant death.

4. moreover/furthermore/in addition

We use these expressions to add information to what has been said. The usage of these words is much more elegant than just making a list or using the conjunction "and".

Examples:

- In the present study, the audiovestibular symptoms were assessed retrospectively and could therefore be biased. *Moreover*, these symptoms were not objectively assessed.
- These results suggest new potential therapeutic biomarkers in lung carcinoma. *Furthermore*, the results of another cDNA microarray study indicate that the overexpression of the tumor-suppressor gene PTEN may inhibit lung cancer invasion by downregulating a panel of genes.
- *In addition to* its more thoroughly studied role in degradation, the autophagic machinery is also involved in a less known process termed secretory autophagy.

5. therefore/as a result/consequently

These expressions show that the second statement follows logically from the first statement.

Examples:

- He reduced the amount of time studying for his final exams. *As a result*, his marks were rather low.
- In this clinical setting, the physician referring to the MPS examination was blinded to the result of the TDE-CFR, which, *consequently*, did not affect or guide the clinical decision process in this experimental study.
- These results demonstrate that the established UPLC method was accurate and precise and *therefore* appropriate for the quantitative analyses.

II. Writing Medical Papers in English

4-Step Approach to Writing the Introduction Section of a Research Paper
By Yateendra Joshi

If you want others to cite your paper, you should make sure they read it first. Let us assume that the title and the abstract of your paper have convinced your peers that they should see your paper. It is then the job of the Introduction section to ensure that they start reading it and keep reading it, to pull them in and to show them around as it were, guiding them to the other parts of the paper (Methods, Results, Discussion, and Conclusion).

This article tells you, with examples, what you should include in the Introduction and what you should leave out, and what reviewers and journal editors look for in this section.

What is the function of the Introduction section?

Put simply, the Introduction should answer the question "Why": why you choose that topic for research; why it is important; why you adopted a particular method or approach; and so on. You can also think of the Introduction as the section that points out the gap in knowledge that the rest of the paper will fill, or the section in which you define and claim your territory within the broad area of research.

The other job the Introduction should do is to give some background information and set the context. You can do this by describing the research problem you considered or the research question you asked (in the main body of the paper, you will offer the solution to the problem or the answer to the question) and by briefly reviewing any other solutions or approaches that have been tried in the past.

Remember that a thesis or a dissertation usually has a separate chapter titled "Review of Literature", but a research paper has no such section; instead, the Introduction includes a review in brief.

Now that you have given the background and set the context, the last part of the Introduction should specify the objectives of the experiment or analysis of the study described in the paper. This concluding part of the Introduction should include specific details or the exact question(s) to be answered later in the paper.

The 4-step approach to writing the Introduction section

As a rule of thumb, this section accounts for about 10% of the total word count of the body of a typical research paper, or about 400 words spread over three paragraphs in a 4000-word paper. With that, let us now understand how to write the Introduction section step-by-step.

1. Provide background information and set the context. This initial part of the Introduction prepares the readers for more detailed and specific information that is given later. The first couple of sentences are typically broad. For example, a paper that discusses the possible beneficial role of bacteria in treating cancer can begin as follows: "The role of bacteria as anticancer agent was recognized almost hundred years back." At the same time, the introductory statement should not be too broad: note that in this example, the Introduction did not begin by talking about cancer by mentioning the role of bacteria.

Once the first sentence has introduced the broad field, the next sentence can point to the specific area within that broad field. As you may have noticed, the paper in the example mentioned above introduced the subfield by mentioning remission of some types cancer following accidental infection by Streptococcus pyogenes.

2. Introduce the specific topic of your research and explain why it is important. As you can see from the above examples, the authors are moving toward presenting the specific topic of their research. So now in the following part, you can bring in some statistics to show the importance of the topic or the seriousness of the problem.

Here are two examples:

Example 1: *A paper on controlling malaria by preventive measures, can mention the number of people affected, the number of person-hours lost, or the cost of treating the disease.*

Example 2: *A paper on developing crops that require little water can mention the frequency of severe droughts or the decrease in crop production because of droughts.*

Another way to emphasize the importance of the research topic is to highlight the possible benefits from solving the problem or from finding an answer to the question: possible savings, greater production, longer-lasting devices, and so on. This approach emphasizes the positive.

For example, instead of saying that X dollars are lost because of malaria every year, say that X dollars can be saved annually if malaria is prevented, or X millions litres of water can be saved by dispensing with irrigation, or X person-hours can be saved in the form of avoided illnesses because of improved air quality or reduced pollution.

3. Mention past attempts to solve the research problem or to answer the research question. As mentioned earlier, a formal review of literature is out of place in the Introduction section of a research paper; however, it is appropriate to indicate any earlier relevant research and clarify how your research differs from those attempts. The differences can be simple: you may have repeated the same set of experiments but with a different organism, or elaborated (involving perhaps more sophisticated or advanced analytical instruments) the study with a much larger and diverse sample, or a widely different geographical setting.

Here are two examples:

Example 3: *Although these studies were valuable, they were undertaken when the draft genome sequence had not been available and therefore provide little information on the evolutionary and regulatory mechanisms.*

Example 4: *Plant response is altered by insect colonization and behaviour but these aspects have been studied mostly in sole crops, whereas the present paper examines the relationship between crops and their pests in an inter-cropping system.*

4. Conclude the Introduction by mentioning the specific objectives of your research. The earlier paragraphs should lead logically to specific objectives of your study. Note that this part of the Introduction gives specific details: for instance, the earlier part of the Introduction may mention the importance of controlling malaria whereas the concluding part will specify what methods of control were used and how they were evaluated. At the same time, avoid too much detail because those belong to the Materials and Methods section of the paper.

Here are two examples:

Example 5: *We aimed to assess the effectiveness of four disinfection strategies on hospital-wide incidence of multidrug-resistant organisms and Clostridium difficile.*

Example 6: *We aimed ① to assess the epidemiological changes before and after the upsurge of scarlet fever in China in 2011; ② to explore the reasons for the upsurge and the epidemiological factors that contributed to it; and ③ to assess how these factors could be managed to prevent future epidemics.*

Besides infinitives as shown in examples in the previous paragraphs, questions and hypotheses may also be used as ways of constructing the objectives:

Questions

Example 7: *Do some genes in wheat form gene networks? If they do, to what extent as compared to rice?*

Example 8: *Do the regulatory elements in the promoters of those genes display any conserved motifs?*

Example 9: *Finally, and more specifically, do those genes in wheat display any tissue- or organ-specific expression pattern?*

Hypotheses

Example 10: *We decided to test the following hypotheses related to employees of information-technology companies:*

H1: Career stages influence work values.

H2: Career stages influence the level of job satisfaction.

H3: Career stages do not influence organizational commitment.

Compared to two other sections of a typical research paper, namely Methods and Results, Introduction and Discussion are more difficult to write. However, the 4-step approach described in this article should ease the task.

A final tip: although the Introduction is the first section of the main text of your paper, you don't have to write that section first. You can write it, or at least revise it, after you have written the rest of the paper: this will make the Introduction not only easier to write but also more compelling.

Unit 5

Medicine and Technology

Task 1 *Watch the video and answer the following questions, and then exchange your answers with your classmates.*

1. Can you explain "Medical care is still a high-touch service" in your own words?

_____

_____

2. According to the conversation, what advantages does AI show on diagnosis?

_____

_____

3. Some holds the view that the doctors will be replaced by AI, do you agree or disagree with such point of view? Please present your reasons.

_____

_____

Task 2 *Watch the video again and fill in the following gaps. Make sure the word(s) you fill in is(are) both grammatically and semantically acceptable.*

Mr Chiang: Historically and experience wise, medical care is still high-touch business, high-touch service. It remains controversial (1) _____.

Anchorwoman (Nancy Hungerford):

—Nothing replaces the human altogether;

—Question: (2) _____?

Mr Chiang:

—A mother of a pair of twins is given as an example;

—One of the twins got (3) _____ while the other _____.

—Suggestion for the situation: (4) _____.

—In terms of treatment, patients need (5) _____.

—AI cannot replace the historical high-touch doctor-patient relationship.

Anchorwoman: Right.

Mr Chiang:

—AI is definitely helpful particularly in (6) _____ and also in (6) _____.

—With the help of AI, patients can (7) _____.

Anchorwoman: And I think the message there is that it's improving health care, but AI is not going to replace the human doctor.

Mr Chiang: I see it's enhancing. Whether it's complementary or not, it's hard to say at this stage.

Anchorwoman: Jai's patients face a little bit of a different scenario in that (8) ____ _____.

Jai Verma:

—We are building a tele-medicine in our APPS today where (9) _____ _____.

—Patients can consult the doctor in the middle of the night through (10) _____ _____.

—AI, internet of things (物联网) are going to change the way we deliver health care in the future.

—With AI we can reduce a lot of medical mistakes and save millions of lives.

Part I Intensive Reading

Ethical Challenges to Use of Artificial Intelligence for Health Care

1 Several ethical challenges are emerging with the use of AI for health, many of which are especially relevant to low- and middle-income countries (LMIC). These challenges must be addressed if AI technologies are to support achievement of universal health coverage. Use of AI to extend health-care coverage and services in marginalized communities in HIC can raise similar ethical concerns, including an enduring digital divide, lack of good-quality data, collection of data that incorporate clinical biases (as well as inappropriate data collection practices) and lack of treatment options after diagnosis.

2 There are risks of overstatement of what AI can accomplish, unrealistic estimates of what could be achieved as AI evolves and uptake of unproven products and services that have not been subjected to rigorous evaluation for safety and efficacy. This is due partly to the enduring appeal of "technological solutionism", in which technologies such as AI are used as a "magic bullet" to remove deeper social, structural, economic and institutional barriers. The appeal of technological solutions and the promise of technology can lead to overestimation of the benefits and **dismissal** of the challenges and problems that new technologies such as AI may introduce. This can result in an unbalanced health-care policy and misguided investments by countries that have few resources and by high-income countries (HIC) that are under pressure to reduce public expenditure on health care. It can also divert attention and resources from proven but underfunded interventions that would reduce morbidity and mortality in LMIC.

3 First, the AI technology itself may not meet the standards of scientific validity and accuracy that are currently applied to medical technologies. For example, digital technologies developed in the early stages of the COVID-19 pandemic did not necessarily meet any objective standard of efficacy to justify their use. AI technologies have been introduced as part of the pandemic response without adequate evidence, such as from randomized clinical trials, or safeguards. An emergency does not justify deployment of unproven technologies; in fact, efforts to ensure that resources were allocated where they were most urgently needed should have heightened the vigilance of both companies and governments (such as regulators and ministries of health) to ensure that the technologies were accurate and effective.

4 Secondly, the benefits of AI may be overestimated when erroneous or overly optimistic assumptions are made about the infrastructure and institutional context in which the technologies will be used and where the intrinsic requirements for use of the technology cannot be met. In some low-income countries, financial resources and information and communication technology infrastructure lag those of HIC, and the significant investments that would be required might discourage use. The quality and availability of data may not be adequate for use of AI, especially in LMIC. There is a danger that poor-quality data will be collected for AI training, which may result in models that predict artefacts in the data instead of actual clinical outcomes. There may also be no data, which, with poor-quality data, could distort the performance of an algorithm, resulting in inaccurate performance, or an AI technology might not be available for a specific population because of insufficient usable data. Additionally, significant investment may be required to make non-uniform data sets collected in LMIC usable. Compilation of data in resource-poor settings is difficult and time-consuming, and the additional burden on community health workers should be considered. Data are unlikely to be available on the most vulnerable or marginalized populations, including those for whom health-care services are lacking, or they might be inaccurate. Data may also be difficult to collect because of language barriers, and mistrust may lead people to provide incorrect or incomplete information. Often, irrelevant data are collected, which can undermine the overall quality of a data set.

5 There may not be appropriate or enforceable regulations, stakeholder participation or oversight, all of which are required to ensure that ethical and legal concerns can be addressed and human rights are not violated. For example, AI technologies may be introduced in countries without up-to-date data protection and confidentiality laws (especially for health-related data) or without the oversight of data protection authorities to rigorously protect confidentiality and the privacy of individuals and communities. Furthermore, regulatory agencies in LMIC may not have the capacity or expertise to assess AI technologies to ensure that systematic errors do not affect diagnosis, surveillance and treatment.

6 Thirdly, there may be enough ethical concern about a use case or a specific AI technology, even if it provides accurate, useful information and insights, to discourage a particular use. An AI technology that can predict which individuals are likely to develop type-2 diabetes or HIV infection could provide benefits to an at-risk individual or community but could also give rise to unnecessary stigmatization of individuals or communities, whose choices and behaviour are questioned or even criminalized, result in over-medicalization of otherwise healthy individuals, create unnecessary stress and anxiety and expose individuals to aggressive marketing by pharmaceutical companies and other for-profit health-care services. Furthermore, certain AI technologies, if not deployed carefully, could exacerbate disparities in health care, including those related to ethnicity, socioeconomic status or gender.

7 Fourthly, like all new heath technologies, even if an AI technology does not trigger an ethics warning, its benefits may not be justified by the extra expense or cost (beyond information and communication technology infrastructure) associated with the procurement, training and technology investment required. Robotic surgery may produce better outcomes, but the opportunity costs associated with the investment must also be considered.

8 Fifthly, enough consideration may not be given to whether an AI technology is appropriate and adapted to the context of LMIC, such as diverse languages and scripts in a country or among countries. Lack of investment in, for example, translation can mean that certain applications do not operate correctly or simply cannot be used by a population. Such lack of foresight points to a wider problem, which is that many AI technologies are designed by and for high-income populations and by individuals or companies with inadequate understanding of the characteristics of the target populations in LMIC.

9 Unrealistic expectations of what AI can achieve may, however, unnecessarily discourage its use. Thus, machines and algorithms (and the data used for algorithms) are expected in the public imagination to be perfect, while humans can make mistakes. Medical professionals might overestimate their ability to perform tasks and ignore or underestimate the value of algorithmic decision tools, for which the challenges can be managed and for which evidence indicates a measurable benefit. Not using the technology could result in avoidable morbidity and mortality, making it blameworthy not to use a certain AI technology, especially if the standard of care is already shifting to its use.

10 Even after an AI technology has been introduced into a health-care system, its impact should be evaluated continuously during its real-world use, as should the performance of an algorithm if it learns from data that are different from its training data. Impact assessments can also guide a decision on use of AI in an area of health before and after its introduction. Assessment of whether to introduce an AI technology in a low-income country or resource-poor setting may lead to a different conclusion from such an assessment in a high-income setting. Risk-benefit calculations that do not favour a specific use of AI in HIC may be interpreted differently for a low-income country that lacks, for example, enough health-care workers to perform certain tasks or which would otherwise forego use of more accurate diagnostic instruments, such that individuals receive inaccurate diagnoses and the wrong treatment.

11 The use of AI to resource-poor contexts should, however, be extended carefully to avoid situations in which large numbers of people receive accurate diagnoses of a health condition but have no access to appropriate treatment. Health-care workers have a duty to provide treatment after testing for and confirmation of disease, and the relatively low cost at which AI diagnostics can be deployed should be accompanied by careful planning to ensure that people are not left without treatment. Prediction tools for anticipating a disease outbreak will have to be complemented by robust surveillance systems and other effective measures.

Words and Expressions

coverage /ˈkʌvərɪdʒ/ n.
the extent to which something deals with something else

marginalize /ˈmɑːdʒɪnəlaɪz/ adj.
(of a person, group, or concept) being treated as insignificant or peripheral

randomize /ˈrændəmaɪz/ v.
to make (a set of items, people, etc.) unpredictable, unsystematic, or random in order or arrangement

allocate /ˈæləkeɪt/ v.
to distribute (resources or duties) for a particular purpose

vigilance /ˈvɪdʒɪləns/ n.
the action or state of keeping careful watch for possible danger or difficulties

erroneous /ɪˈrəʊniəs/ adj.
(of beliefs, opinions, or methods) being incorrect or only partly correct

infrastructure /ˈɪnfrəstrʌktʃə/ n.
the basic physical and organizational structures and facilities (e.g. buildings, roads, power supplies) needed for the operation of a society or enterprise

intrinsic /ɪnˈtrɪnsɪk/ adj.
belonging naturally; essential

artefact /ˈɑːtɪfækt/ n.
something made or given shape by humankind, such as a tool or a work of art; a spurious experimental result

algorithm /ˈælgərɪðəm/ n.
a set of rules for solving a problem in a finite number of steps, as for finding the greatest common divisor

surveillance /sɜːˈveɪləns/ n.
close observation, especially of a suspected spy or criminal

stigmatization /ˌstɪgmətaɪˈzeɪʃn/ n.
the action of describing or regarding someone or something as worthy of disgrace or great disapproval

pharmaceutical /ˌfɑːməˈsuːtɪkl/ adj.
relating to medicinal drugs, or their preparation, use, or sale

exacerbate /ɪgˈzæsəbeɪt/ v.
to make something that is already bad even worse

procurement /prəˈkjʊəmənt/ n.
the act of obtaining or acquiring sth.

I. Reading Comprehension

Choose the best answer to each of the following questions.

1. The ethical challenges that rise with the application of AI in medical field do NOT include _____ .

   A. unfitting data collection approach

   B. proper therapeutic methods after diagnosis

   C. absence of qualified data

   D. durable digital gap

2. According to the author, a series of factors except the _____ of the AI technology should be assessed before AI is put into practice.

   A. precision　　B. moral codes　　C. privacy　　　D. pattern

3. The word "dismissal" in Paragraph 2 has the meaning of _____ .

   A. furlough　　B. discharge　　C. redundancy　　D. avoidance

4. Which of the following statement is true?

   A. The functions of AI tend to be underestimated.

   B. The expenditure of AI is a little high currently.

   C. LMIC appear to be in the lead in AI application.

   D. HIC are standing a better chance in tackling ethical challenges.

5. The author adopts _____ tone on AI technology.

   A. an exaggerated　　　　　B. an emotional

   C. a matter-of-fact　　　　　D. a pessimistic

II. Vocabulary

Task 1　*Fill in the blanks of the following sentences with the words or expressions given in the box below. Change the forms where necessary.*

trigger	algorithm	allocated	marginalize	surveillance
pharmaceutical	vigilance	intrinsic	erroneous	randomized
stigmatization	artefact	infrastructure	coverage	procurement

1. The order in which the trials were presented was _____ separately for each participant.

2. The sensor is connected via a computer _____ to an insulin pump which administers doses of the hormone automatically when required.

3. If people are healthy and educated they are then stronger to improve their own

communities and build sound _____ .

4. The effect of this has been to increasingly _____ the local authority sector.

5. In patients with autoimmune diseases, however, UV light may _____ inflammatory responses.

6. It is the degree and extent of its _____ of a part of a building which translates a mere fixing into a fitting.

7. If public bodies continue to exclude local firms from their _____ process, all the brave words about a Smart Successful Scotland will ring hollow.

8. Vaccinations are limited and will be _____ to those who apply first.

9. We performed two experiments in order to eliminate the possibility that the recombination we observed was an _____ of the PCR reaction.

10. It is also required to maintain constant _____ against external threats to the integrity and vitality of the body.

11. Police have been monitoring the site and using covert _____ to trap the troublemakers.

12. They did nothing to dispel his _____ belief about the children's paternity.

13. He argues that the world will only get better at dealing with addiction once addicts can speak without fear of _____ .

14. It is open to the general public and aims to underline the _____ value of the subject as a core life skill.

15. The organisation believes that the _____ industry is willing to lower the price of antimalarial drugs.

Task 2) *Under each of the following boxes there are several groups of sentences. In each sentence a common word or expression is missing. Find it out from the corresponding box according to the meaning and structure of the sentences. The forms of the words and expressions may change in the sentences.*

efficacy	mortality	morbidity	validity

Group 1

1. The heptavalent vaccine seems to have modest protective _____ against otitis media, the illness accounting for most antibiotic use in children.

2. A steroid injection is thought to combine the _____ of oral steroids with the limited side effect profile of topical steroids and is typically performed in the clinic setting.

3. Given this finding and the lack of previous safety and _____ data, we sought to test the effects of PCC under conditions replicating a hemorrhagic shock-associated coagulopathy with the presence of severe metabolic acidosis.

Answer: _____

Group 2

1. Left ventricular enlargement is known to be a strong predictor of _____ and death from coronary heart disease independent of its association with raised systolic blood pressure and increased body mass.

2. Postoperative _____ and hospitalisation were significantly less with ESWL and endourological procedures than with other open surgical techniques.

3. Chronic mucus hypersecretion (CMH) is a common symptom in patients suffering from asthma, especially patients with more severe or poorly controlled disease, and this respiratory symptom is now considered to be a risk factor for increased _____ in patients suffering from asthma.

Answer: _____

Group 3

1. In examining the construct _____ of the results, logistic regression was first used to explore the explanatory factors that people gave for stating either yes or no to the starting point WTP bid.

2. Furthermore, despite the wide scope and established _____ of this database, coding accuracy and consistency of data collected are dependent on coding expertise and experience.

3. Similar to McCormac's methodology, we assumed the of the _____ at the onset of the study based on previous work including normal subjects and patients with schizophrenia and schizoaffective disorder.

Answer: _____

Group 4

1. Despite recent advances in clinical cancer treatment strategies, such as chemotherapy and immunotherapy, the oral cancer is the second leading cause of cancer-related _____.

2. An unadjusted logistic regression model was used to estimate the OR for inpatient _____ among patients with CS relative to quartiles of volume for CS.

3. In contrast, for a 50-year-old woman who has smoked since adolescence and does not stop, a 55% increase in the lung cancer _____ rate would change her risk of death from lung cancer before age 80 years from approximately 9.4% to 13.8%.

Answer: _____

| uptake   expertise   assumption   emerge |

Group 5

1. Although many of the cosmetic, quality of life, and functional improvements have been proved, a better understanding of the procedure and the appropriate indications for its application will continue to develop even as the technique itself evolves, and as new approaches _____.

2. In the same way, results of studies carry different inherent credibility because they _____ from different study designs.

3. If the hydrophobic handoff model turns out to be correct, it still leaves a major problem: how does the cholesterol move from the NTD of NPC1 to enter the membrane and _____ on the other side for transport to the ER and plasma membrane?

Answer: _____

Group 6

1. We tested this _____ and found no evidence of differential pre-trends for all payer share outcome variables except a small differential trend for the uninsured share of surgical discharges in small expansion states.

2. Magnetic susceptibility was referenced (0 ppb) to the average susceptibility of the brain, with the _____ that a larger reference region would reduce additional interparticipant variability compared with a smaller reference region.

3. The lack of correlation between these features does not support this _____.

Answer: _____

Group 7

1. The liver handles glucose bidirectionally, that is, both by _____ and by release.

2. In addition, patients with high-grade infiltration had significantly higher levels of gadolinium _____ compared with patients who had low-grade infiltration.

3. The finding indicates a pulmonary _____ of cadmium in the studied children with asthma from direct inhalation of side stream smoke from their parents' cigarettes.

Answer: _____

Group 8

1. All of these factors, in addition to the improvement in the technical _____ of endourological surgeons, have contributed to a significant decline in the current indications for open stone surgery.

2. Thus，the clinician practicing EBM may need to be able to apply his or her _____ in different ways，depending on the clinical scenario.

3. For a query that is well studied and a patient who is dissimilar to those who were in those studies，clinician _____ requires a more discerning role to weigh the potentially different，patient-specific risks and benefits.

Answer：_____

III. **Cloze**

Fill in each of the following blanks with the most appropriate word from each of the four choices given.

Promoting the use of big data in medicine is a national priority in China. In June 2016，the State Council of China ___1___ an official notice on the development，and use of big data in the healthcare sector. The council acknowledged that big data in health and medicine were a strategic national resource and their development could ___2___ healthcare in China，and it set out programmatic development goals，key tasks，and an organisational framework.

After regional health data centres were ___3___ in Shanghai and Ningbo，the National Health and Family Planning Commission announced in 2016 that China would establish more regional and national centres and industrial parks that focused on big data in health and medicine as part of a national ___4___ programme to make more meaningful use of these data. Four cities in Fujian and Jiangsu provinces in eastern China were chosen as the pilot sites，and the centres are now in construction.

China is already making use of big data. The country's personal identification system could be used to link data from various sources. Medical ___5___ data from the national social insurance system have been used to generate a 5% sampling database and an overall database covering over 0.6 billion beneficiaries in the past five years，which are ___6___ to scientific researchers.

Applications to use these data are managed by organisations such as the Chinese Health Insurance Research Association；there is no public ___7___ . Since 2016，many academic research projects using these national datasets have been ___8___ to evaluate the current and future clinical and economic burden of ___9___ diseases such as cardiovascular disease，diabetes，kidney disease，and chronic obstructive pulmonary disease. Furthermore，other national administrative databases，including the national standardised discharge summary of inpatients and the national death registry，with hundreds of millions of patient records，have been used by medical and public health researchers.

China is also focusing on personalising medicine. Since 2016, the Ministry of Science and Technology has __10__ and funded many "precision medicine" projects under the national key research and development programme. A centralised and integrated data __11__ for precision medicine is being developed, which will store all patient/population data as well as biosamples collected from a series of large cohort studies and from biobanks. The platform is __12__ to include at least 0.7 million participants, 0.4 million from the general population and 0.3 million from patients with major non-communicable diseases. China's large population base and centralised governance mean that very large sample sizes can be reached, which is of great value to __13__ medicine initiatives.

As well as the government-led projects, Chinese academic medical societies are __14__ data-sharing initiatives. In October 2017, the School of Public Health at Peking University __15__ the launch of the China Cohort Consortium. Currently 20 cohorts with more than 2 million participants are included.

1. A. pressed   B. issued   C. announced   D. declared
2. A. cultivate   B. develop   C. improve   D. facilitate
3. A. established   B. built   C. created   D. erected
4. A. probing   B. investigational C. experimental   D. pilot
5. A. claims   B. admits   C. assets   D. affirms
6. A. suitable   B. identifiable   C. reliable   D. available
7. A. entrance   B. access   C. path   D. approach
8. A. assigned   B. granted   C. approved   D. assisted
9. A. chronic   B. acute   C. malignant   D. benignant
10. A. advocated   B. encouraged   C. initiated   D. originated
11. A. collection   B. platform   C. processing   D. analyzing
12. A. expected   B. intended   C. programmed   D. organized
13. A. averaged   B. specialized   C. routinized   D. personalized
14. A. contributing B. leading   C. absenting   D. presenting
15. A. announced   B. broadcasted   C. published   D. condemned

IV. Discussion and Presentation

Answer the following questions on the basis of your reading.

1. What functions does AI serve in the fight against COVID-19?

2. Except for the ethical challenges which are mentioned in the passage，are there any other moral problems emerging from the application of AI technology in clinical practice?

3. Would you please present some specific examples to illustrate "the use of AI in LMIC should be very cautious"?

V. Translation

Translate the following sentences into English.

1. 新冠病毒（COVID-19）的教训之一是，世界需要在数据分析方面取得重大进步，以帮助领导人做出明智的公共卫生决策。

   _____

2. 像所有新技术一样，人工智能在改善世界各地数以百万计的人的健康方面具有巨大潜力，但像所有技术一样，人工智能也可能被滥用并造成伤害。

   _____

4. 人工智能可以让患者更好地掌控自己的卫生保健，更好地了解自己不断变化的需求。

   _____

4. 随着越来越多的国家、公司和个人开始使用数字技术应对新冠病毒的影响，有韧性且值得信赖的电信网络和服务必不可少。

   _____

5. 我国在健康和医疗领域全国性推广使用大数据，在不久的将来，这将在很大程度上改变我国现有的医学研究和医疗实践手段，促进医疗保健行业的发展。

   _____

VI. Further Readings

1. Risk，Benefit，and Fairness in a Big Data World

2. A Review of Big Data and Medical Research

3. The WHO Guidance on Ethics & Governance of Artificial Intelligence for Health

Part II   Academic Development

I. Translating Medical Texts

Read the following sample abstract and put the underlined part into English.

【摘要】人工智能技术的快速发展,得益于大数据、数据库、算法、算力的巨大进步,<u>医学研究是人工智能的重要应用方向。人工智能与医学的融合发展,提高了医疗技术水平与医疗服务效率,为医生与医疗设备有效赋能,更好地服务于患者。特别在此次新冠肺炎疫情中取得的巨大成效,足见人工智能在医疗领域中发挥着巨大作用,因此吸引了许多研究者不断深入探索。</u>本文对近年来人工智能在医学方面应用的相关文献进行梳理,基于人工智能技术与医学研究的发展背景,重点论述人工智能在药物研发、辅助诊疗、语音识别和语义理解、健康管理、医院管理等领域的应用进展,分析人工智能在医疗领域应用中存在的挑战,最后讨论人工智能在医疗领域的发展趋势。①

Translation & Writing Skills：Literal Translation

Literal translation is also called direct translation or close translation. It is a method to render text from one language to another by following closely the form of the source language. Using this method，the image，figure of speech，word order，grammatical structure，etc. of the source language are maintained in the target language.

Examples：

摊牌	to show one's cards
武装到牙齿	to be armed to the teeth
掉鳄鱼眼泪	to shed crocodile tears
以眼还眼,以牙还牙	an eye for an eye, a tooth for a tooth

However，we need to bear in mind that literal translation is not rigid translation（死译）or word-for-word translation（逐字翻译）. Now let's compare：

干预措施主要包括：<u>发挥家庭和同伴支持的作用,定期电话随访、门诊随访和知识讲座。</u>

Version 1：to play the role of family and peer support，regular telephone follow-up, out-patient follow-up and knowledge lectures.（×）

Version 2：giving full play to family and peer support，making regular telephone follow-up，outpatient follow-up and delivering health lectures.（√）

---

① 选自《中国医学物理学杂志》2021 年第 8 期,1044 - 1047 页。作者:巩高、黄文华、曹石、陈超敏、郑东宏。

The first version uses word-for-word translation，which sounds quite ridiculous. The second version makes proper adaption，yet conveys the meaning of the original sentence more faithfully and clearly.

More Examples：

1. 纸厂通常会在现场蒸煮原淀粉(即未改性淀粉)或改性淀粉以备使用。

Paper mills normally cook native（unmodified）or modified starch onsite to prepare it for use.

2. 双击此图标测试双击设置。如果此图标不发生变化,则使用以上网格调整设置。

Double-click this icon to test your double-click settings. If this icon doesn't change，adjust your settings using the grid above.

3. 医疗机器人在医疗活动中的广泛应用极大地推动了医学的发展。

The extensive application of medical robots in medical activities has greatly promoted the development of medicine.

4. 增加膳食钙、补充钙剂(联合或不联合维生素 D)对青少年的骨密度、骨峰值有一定的有益作用,可以延缓老年人群的骨量流失,但对青少年成年后的身高、增加成人的骨密度以及预防老年人群的骨折并无明显作用。

Increasing dietary calcium and supplementing calcium（with or without vitamin D）have a certain beneficial effect on the bone mineral density and its peak of adolescents and can delay the bone loss of the elderly，but it can't improve the height and bone mineral density of adults or prevent fracture in the elderly.

II. Writing Medical Papers in English

General Considerations for Materials and Methods Section
By Asghar Ghasemi，et al .

The Materials and Methods section of a scientific paper is a crossroads connecting the introduction to the results section to create a clear story line；it should clearly present the approach to answer the main study question(s)，i. e. questions like who，what，where，when，why，and how. We could also refer to this section as the Experimental section，Method Description and Validation，or Patients/Subjects and Methods. In this review specific recommendations will be provided regarding the M&M section of clinical，experimental，epidemiological，and genetic studies.

1. Length

Typical length of the M&M section is 2-3 pages, consisting of 6-9 paragraphs (each paragraph usually contains 100 - 200 words, not exceeding 750 words); however, depending on the discipline and field of study, the length of this section may vary from the condensed to the extended form. Method sections of chemistry, mycology, and molecular biology may be categorized as condensed-form, whereas public health and medical research are considered as intermediate, and psychology, sociology, and education are organized in the extended-form. To keep the M&M more concise, some details of materials and methods may be allowed as appendix or supplementary documents that are published online.

To organize paragraphs, topic sentences can be used to signal the topic of a paragraph, especially when a subsection has more than one paragraph. The use of linking or transition phrases/clauses (purpose phrases, time-related linking phrases, or causal linking phrases) to signal the topic of a paragraph is highly recommended (Table 1).

2. Tables and Figures in Methods: Yes or No?

The use of appropriate tables and figures helps authors to summarize large amounts of complex information of the study procedures; a common recommendation to reduce the word count. Flowchart of the study design may be a common form of figure referenced within the M&M section. Some guidelines are available to organize study flowcharts for different study designs, for instance, the CONSORT flow diagram for clinical trials and the STROBE flowchart of study participants for observational designs like cohort studies. This section does not include results, although intermediate results such those used for calculations that are used for obtaining results for the study question such as standard curves are recommended to be included in this section.

Table 1 Useful Phrases to Organize Paragraphs of Methods Section

Aim	Phrases/Clauses
To state purpose of method (purpose phrases at the beginning of a sentence)	to detect, to avoid, in order to identify/understand, to enable, to allow, to determine, to control, to establish whether, to compare, in an attempt to make
To link related-time procedures	before, after, during, prior to, on arrival
To state a reason (causal related phrases)	Based on, on the basis, because of, in spite of, in light of
To justify the use of a special method	we believe, we think

Aim	Phrases/Clauses
To state similarity with previous methods	is reported, is detailed, as described, as explained, as proposed, is based on, was inspired by, is practically the same
To describe the apparatus and materials	use, adopt, employ, consists of, is made up of, is composed of, is based on, design, develop, set up, incorporate, exploit

3. Ordering Procedures in the Materials and Methods Section

Several parts of the M&M section should be written in a logical or chronological order; presenting the methods in a logical order helps the text to make complete sense; however, the actions should be mentioned in chronological order within a paragraph or sentence. Some believe that the use of numbers or bullets to describe a sequential procedure, provided that it is acceptable by the journal, makes the M&M section easier to read. As a general suggestion, no more than two actions should be presented in a sentence. To increase readability, the subject and verb in a sentence should preferably be close together.

4. Tenses and Voices

A general recommendation is that the M&M section should be written in the past tense, either in active or passive voice. Depending on the author's field, the journal style, or the action described in the M&M section, the present simple tense may also be used, for example, this tense is required when a standard method is described or when the authors present their procedure, model, software, or device.

Although passive voice (e. g. *was/were investigated*, *was/were evaluated*, or w*as/were performed*) is the more common form of verbs in this section, using the active voice to show the ownership of the investigators (e. g. *we performed*, *we evaluated*, or *we implemented*) have recently taken priority. However, there is a belief that the active voice is not appropriate for the M&M section because the focus would be shifted from the research to the researchers.

5. Self-Assessing the Quality of the Materials and Methods Section

Self-assessment of the quality of the M&M section may be the last, but it is certainly not the least important step in the writing of the M&M section. Authors need to ask themselves "would a researcher be able to reproduce the study with the information provided in the method section?". Using this approach, the authors would be reassured that all the critical information has been included, and unnecessary and redundant data have been excluded from this section; this process is useful to keep the paper's storyline. In Table 2, a checklist comprised of the most important questions for general quality assessment of the Methods section is provided.

To ensure all the necessary information is included in the Methods section, referring to reporting guidelines that are available for the most common study types (e.g. CONSORT for clinical trials, STROBE for observational studies, STARD for diagnostic research, PRISMA for systematic reviews and meta-analyses, and ARRIVE for animal studies) is highly recommended.

Table 2   Most Important Questions for Self-Assessment of the Methods Section

Questions
Does the method describe the procedures such that reader can easily follow and replicate it?
Is the length of the Methods section (number of paragraphs and sentences) appropriate?
Are the subheadings and paragraphs appropriately organized?
Has every step been covered in a clear and complete manner?
Has choosing of the method been clearly justified?
Is the method as concise as possible, with clear and short sentences?
Have the previous methods been properly cited?
Has everything been provided in a logical and/or chronological order?
Have linking phrases (purpose statements, time-related phrases, justifying phrases) been properly used?
Does the Methods section meet the grammatical constructions correctly?
Have the correct tenses (past simple vs. present simple) been used throughout the text?
Have abbreviations been used minimally and in a proper and reasonable way? (Use standard abbreviations instead of writing complete words; define each abbreviation the first time that it is used)
Has the Methods section been organized according to the journal's style?

The M&M section is the most important part of a research paper because it provides detailed information to other scientists/researchers to reproduce the study and judge the validity of the study's findings. In the M&M section, "materials" refers to what was examined (e.g. humans, animals, cell lines, or tissues) and various chemicals and treatments (e.g. drugs, culture media, and gases), and the instruments used in the study. "Methods" presents how subjects or objects were employed to answer the study question, that is, how measurements and calculations were made and how data analysis was carried out. Useful tips and common pitfalls in the M&M section are briefly reviewed in Table 3.

Table 3　Brief Review of Useful Tips and Common Pitfalls in the Materials and Methods Section

Useful tips	Common pitfalls
√ Describe the study design, setting and participants, data collection, data analysis, and ethics approval √ Keep a logical or chronological order in writing √ Provide values for the number of patients, animals, or the number of cells, organs, and biopsies for in vitro study √ Provide inclusion and exclusion criteria of the subjects √ Describe details for recruitment of the study subjects, randomization and/or blinding √ In case of intervention, provide dose, administration route, timing of administration, duration of intervention √ Provide exact information about the control group (e. g. placebo, saline, vehicle) √ Describe primary, secondary, and other outcomes √ Describe details of the measurements √ Describe validity and reliability of measurement tools	❖ Too little or too much information ❖ Lack of providing method for all results ❖ Use of "dangling modifier" because of over-reliance on passive voice ❖ Lack of approval by an institutional review board ❖ Lack of approval by the ethics research committee ❖ Inappropriate, sub-optimal, insufficiently described instrument ❖ Insufficient description of study population ❖ Incomplete description of the sampling method ❖ Lack of adequacy in addressing confounding variables ❖ Describing methods like an advertisement

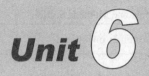

Unit 6

Life and Death

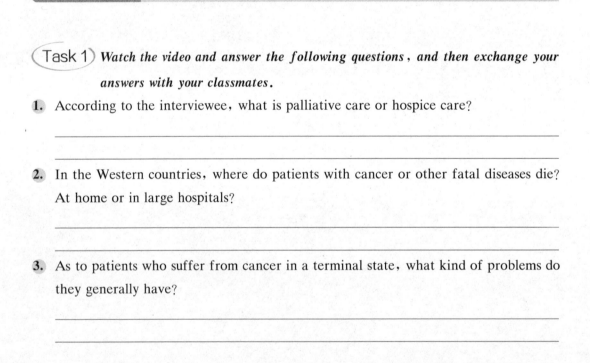

Lead-in : Chinese Government Published Guidelines on the Construction of Hospice Centers

(Task 1) *Watch the video and answer the following questions, and then exchange your answers with your classmates.*

1. According to the interviewee, what is palliative care or hospice care?

   _____

   _____

2. In the Western countries, where do patients with cancer or other fatal diseases die? At home or in large hospitals?

   _____

   _____

3. As to patients who suffer from cancer in a terminal state, what kind of problems do they generally have?

   _____

   _____

(Task 2) *Watch the video again and fill in the following gaps. Make sure the word(s) you fill in is(are) both grammatically and semantically acceptable.*

   Li Xiaomei from Oncology Department of the PLA General Hospital shared 2 points about the news that the Chinese government had published guidelines on the

096

administration of hospice care.

The first point is that the publishing releases a very clear message that (1) _____
_____ . The second point is that it encourages
(2) _____ since patients with terminal illness face many problems.

Many consensuses have been made concerning hospice care during the past 30 years
but they are largely limited to (3) _____ . The significance of publishing
these guidelines lies in the fact that hospice care have (4) _____ from our
government.

The reasons for the slow development of hospice care in China are of two
folds. The first is the lack of (5) _____ among medical professionals. The
second should be the (6) _____ .

The cost of hospice care is not really a big problem because that amount is
reimbursed by the (7) _____ .

The main reasons for low international ranking in terms of hospice service include
lack of (8) _____ and (9) _____ .

Part I　Intensive Reading

Hospice and Palliative Care in China: Development and Challenges
By Yuhan Lu, Youhui Gu, Wenhua Yu

1 Hospice care is end-of-life care provided by health professionals and volunteers
who give medical, psychological, and spiritual support to dying patients and their
families. The goal is to help people who are dying live their last days peacefully and with
dignity. Palliative care is a caring approach through prevention, assessment, and
treatment of pain and other physical, psychological, or spiritual problems, which
improves the quality of life of patients and their families facing life-threatening
illness. Hospice and palliative care has been demonstrated to improve quality of life,
reduce costs, and shorten hospital stays.

Context of Care in China

2 The ageing population and the growing number of patients with cancer in China
have led to the increasing need for hospice and palliative care service.

3 Hospice and palliative care as a specialty in China was first started by experts
from medical facilities and academic associations. In some specialized cancer hospitals,
teams composed of medical professionals began working in inpatient and outpatient

services. In 1994, the Committee of Rehabilitation and Palliative Care (CRPC) of China Anti-cancer Association was founded. It achieves its mission by supporting research, promoting education and training, and improving public awareness. Experts in the association, such as physicians, nurses, and psychotherapists from different hospitals have led the implementation of hospice and palliative care services within medical facilities where there is the most urgent need for hospice and palliative care.

4 Hospice and palliative care services are provided in various forms in China: inpatient specialized units, inpatient specialized beds, outpatient units, and home care. The inpatient specialized unit takes one of the hospital units as a hospice or palliative care unit. Inpatient specialized beds involve assigning several independent beds in a unit as specialized hospice care beds. However, in both units, the provision of care is often carried out by interdisciplinary teams composed of specially trained professionals working in their hospitals. In outpatient services, consultation about and support for symptom management and emergency conditions is provided. Home care is usually provided by primary medical facilities such as community hospitals and health clinics.

Development of Hospice and Palliative Care

Government Policy and Approach

5 With the promotion by CRPC, in 2011, the National Health and Family Planning Commission (NHFPC) of the People's Republic of China initiated a national program to establish pilot units for standard management for cancer patients with pain in general and specialized hospitals. More than 735 pilot units were established as models providing a conceptual framework to facilitate consistency in the development and distribution of palliative care services for pain management across China by October 2015, and the number reached 913 in 2017.

6 The NHFPC, in February 2017, released three documents on hospice care. These documents stipulate the standards of structure, human resource, and environment of the hospice care service with quality monitoring standards and practice guidelines for health caregivers. The presence of these documents has further accelerated the development of the hospice care service in China. At the same time, the government also initiated a plan to establish five national pilot hospice and palliative care programs in big cities such as Beijing, Shanghai, Changchun, and others.

Medication Availability

7 Owing to the dedication of the CRPC, the most widely used medication for pain relief and many other essential palliative medicines have been covered by medical insurance in accordance with the WHO list of essential palliative medicines. To ensure enough opioids for medical use for patients with pain, the State Council of China issued

the *Regulations on Narcotic Drugs and Psychotropic Substances* in 2005. As a result of a mandate that NHFPC was released, detailed rules and administrative measures for prescription of analgesics were formulated to ensure the medication was available for the treatment. These efforts have promoted opioid availability for patients suffering from cancer pain.

Education for Health Providers

8 Since the establishment of the CRPC, various educational opportunities such as seminars, workshops, and conferences, have emerged across China. These educational offerings have effectively advanced the specialization of palliative care throughout China. In some specialized hospitals, palliative care has become a part of continuing education courses that are easily available for doctors and nurses.

9 In 2009, the Chinese Nurses Association recognized the apparent need and began to offer educational opportunities in hospice and palliative care in their certification course for oncology nurses. The content consisted of 14 class hours divided into six modules, namely, nursing care at the end of life, pain and other symptoms management, communication, ethical issues, spiritual care, and grief and bereavement. In the past 9 years, 1,797 nurses have attended the education course "Certificated Oncology Nurse" for end-of-life care.

Patient Education and Public Advocacy

10 There are many public education programs across China. Five years ago, nurses at Beijing Cancer Hospital initiated an education program called "The Pain Education Program" for patients suffering from cancer pain. Patients learned to take the pain relief medication accurately and clarify their concerns about opioids. Within the same period, over 1,600 patients and family members attended various health education programs in the hospital. In 2016, a caregiver education program for family members called "Warmth with You" was implemented. This program educates family members about how to care for their loved ones, deal with emotions, talk about dying and death, respect the patients' right of knowing the truth, and make decisions.

11 Meanwhile, there are many nonprofit organizations devoted to public advocacy for hospice care. The Chinese Association for Life Care, which was founded in 2006, focuses on caring for the elderly, public welfare, volunteer training, and so on. The Beijing Living Will Promotion Association was founded in 2013, calling for death with dignity by promoting living wills. These organizations have done a lot in promoting the public education for hospice care through websites, journals, activities, training courses, and so on.

Current Issues and Challenges

12 While significant progress has been made in China, China's health-care system still faces many challenges that need to be addressed to ensure that more and more people can benefit from hospice and palliative care service.

Limited Facilities to Offer Hospice and Palliative Care

13 Although many facilities providing various forms of hospice and palliative care services in many provinces have been established during the past decades, none of these forms are widespread or integrated into the mainstream health-care system. The number of facilities is far from meeting the growing demand for hospice and palliative care services, as the population is ageing and the number of patients with life-threatening diseases is increasing in China. For now, most of the hospice and palliative care services are still provided in secondary and tertiary hospitals where high-quality care is provided, while beds for hospice and palliative care are in great shortage.

Essential Medicines for Palliative Care

14 As for the medication availability, pain relief medication in large hospitals and specialized hospitals, such as cancer hospitals, are easily available, while many patients who live in rural and remote communities have limited or no access to opioids. Although a government policy about increasing access to palliative care has ensured that the medication is available, the operating mechanism and monitoring regulations need to be put in place to achieve this goal.

Educational Challenges

15 The rising demand for hospice and palliative care requires more skilled and knowledgeable medical professionals. Thus, training and education need to be continuously supported. Although efforts to improve educational opportunities are in place, implementation of training and education varies between schools of nursing and hospitals, creating inconsistencies in training outcomes. In some nursing schools, the concepts of palliative and hospice care are still integrated into other established courses such as geriatrics nursing and community nursing. In some specialized hospitals, the courses on palliative care are provided through institutional education for all nurses, but this practice is not widely adopted in Chinese hospitals, especially in the remote, rural areas.

Cultural Challenges

16 Although death is believed to be a natural part of life, the Chinese find it hard to think and talk about death and dying, as it may create imbalance in the inner harmony. Further, in China, there is a misunderstanding about the role of palliative and hospice care. Many people have a misconception that once they are offered palliative and hospice care, it means that the health-care providers are giving up them and that they are just waiting for death. They do not want to be regarded as dying persons. As a result, many terminally ill patients refuse the service. Second, diseases and death are inevitable, and they are necessities of life, but most people are reluctant to face them. In some situations when cure is impossible, active treatments, including life-sustaining measures, are still given, which not only increases the patient's suffering but also potentially leads to an undignified death.

17 What's more, in most instances, it is the family members, rather than patients, who usually make decisions; and often, the patients are not included in discussions related to their care. This practice causes patients' confusion and misunderstanding about their illness and prognosis. Many patients have no time to say goodbye, and leave the world with regrets, which does not serve the best interest of the patients or their families.

Words and Expressions

hospice /ˈhɒspɪs/ *n*.
a nursing home that specializes in caring for the terminally ill

palliative /ˈpæliətɪv/ *adj*.
(of a medicine or medical care) relieving pain without dealing with the cause of the condition

specialty /ˈspeʃəlti/ *n*.
a special pursuit, occupation, aptitude, or skill

facility /fəˈsɪləti/ *n*.
a building or place that provides a particular service or is used for a particular industry

rehabilitation /ˌriːəˌbɪlɪˈteɪʃn/ *n*.
restoration to good health or useful life, as through therapy and education

interdisciplinary /ˌɪntədɪsəˈplɪnəri/ *adj*.
of, relating to, or involving two or more academic disciplines that are usually considered distinct

consistency /kənˈsɪstənsi/ *n*.
agreement or logical coherence among things or parts

stipulate /ˈstɪpjuleɪt/ *v*.
to specify or agree to as a condition in an agreement; to concede for the purposes of argument

accelerate /əkˈseləreɪt/ *v*.
to hasten the occurrence of; to increase the speed of

availability /əˌveɪləˈbɪləti/ *n*.
the quality of being at hand when needed; the

opioid /əʊˈpiːəʊɪd/ *n*.
quality of being able to be used or obtained (biochemistry) a compound resembling opium in addictive properties or physiological effects; any of a group of substances that resemble morphine in their physiological or pharmacological effects, esp. in their pain-relieving properties

medication /ˌmedɪˈkeɪʃn/ *n*.
a drug or other form of medicine that is used to treat or prevent disease; the act or process of treating a patient with medicines or remedies

mandate /ˈmændeɪt/ *n*.
an authoritative command or instruction; a command or authorization given by a political electorate to the winner of an election

analgesic /ˌænəlˈdʒiːzɪk/ *adj.* *n*.
(of a drug) acting to relieve pain; a medication that reduces or eliminates pain; a remedy that relieves or allays pain

seminar /ˈsemɪnɑː/ *n*.
a conference or other meeting for discussion or training; any group or meeting for holding discussions or exchanging information

bereavement /bɪˈriːvmənt/ *n*.
state of sorrow over the death or departure of a loved one; the condition of having been deprived of something or someone valued, esp through death

advocacy /ˈædvəkəsi/ *n*.
active support of an idea or cause, etc.; especially the act of pleading or arguing for something; public support for or recommendation of a particular cause or policy

I. Reading Comprehension

Choose the best answer to each of the following questions.

1. Hospice and palliative care has been demonstrated to achieve the following purposes EXCEPT _____ .

   A. improving quality of life   B. prolonging life-span

   C. saving costs   D. shortening hospital stays

2. This article does NOT discuss _____ .

   A. the context of health care in China

   B. the progress China has made during the past decades in hospice and

palliative care

C. the high cost of hospice and palliative care

D. the challenges that will be confronted in the future

3. What does "accelerate" mean in "The presence of these documents further accelerated the development of the hospice care service in China." in Paragraph 6?

   A. Improve.   B. Speed up.   C. Encourage.   D. Initiate.

4. Why do many terminally ill patients refuse hospice and palliative care?

   A. Because they have a misconception towards hospice and palliative care.

   B. Because they believe that death is a natural part of life.

   C. Because they believe that disease and death are inevitable.

   D. Because they believe that hospice and palliative care will lead to an undignified death.

5. Which of the following is NOT TRUE?

   A. Nowadays, the most widely used medication for pain relief and many other essential palliative medicines have been covered by medical insurance.

   B. With the development of hospice and palliative care in China, the schools of nursing lay much emphasis on educating would-be nurses.

   C. End-of-life care has also been covered in hospice and palliative care.

   D. As to the increasing need of hospice and palliative care, China's health-care system faces many challenges.

II. Vocabulary

(Task 1) *Fill in the blanks of the following sentences with the words or expressions given in the box below. Change the forms where necessary.*

initiate	stipulate	accelerate	mandate	available
seminar	bereave	advocacy	inconsistent	specialty
facility	vary	analgesic	multidisciplinary	dignify

1. Symptoms _____ over time as a patient passes through different stages of the disease.

2. Codeine, morphine, and fentanyl were the _____ used most often.

3. Now most diabetics take human insulin made, not in humans, but made in micro-organisms that are growing in a manufacturing _____.

4. Healthcare providers including experts, nurses and other medical workers are all trained to make sure to treat every patient with _____ and respect.

5. His _____ is oncology—working with children with cancer.

6. This programme is to help people to come to terms with loss through _____ or separation.

7. He was cited for his knowledge and skills and his _____ to his fellow doctors in caring for mutual patients.

8. The _____ is aimed at students and those interested in careers in these dynamic sectors.

9. Data mining is a _____ field with many techniques.

10. Neither side believes that it can win a popular _____ for its policies fight things out in an open and honest form.

11. Among the requirements is an agreement _____ the areas of collaboration between the foreign design firm and its mainland counterpart.

12. Civic awareness can take a number of forms, from _____ of a democratic constitution to worker education.

13. Doctors have _____ a series of tests to determine the cause of the problem.

14. The rate of advance of biotech is likely to _____ to such an extent that many people who are alive right now will live to see aeging become at first partially reversible.

15. The evidence given in court was _____ with what he had previously told them.

Task 2 *Under each of the following boxes there are sevral groups of sentences. In each sentence a common word or expression is missing. Find it out from the corresponding box according to the meaning and structure of the sentences. The forms of the words and expressions may change in the sentences.*

challenge analgesic medication accelerate

Group 1

1. In Turkish folk medicine, for example, some Trifolium species are used for their expectorant, _____ , antiseptic properties and are also used to treat rheumatic aches.

2. It should be emphasized that in contrast to the previous trials, our study has evaluated the analgesic effect of magnesium by both subjective variables (VAS, duration of _____ and morphine needed over 48 h) and objective variables (spirometric measurements) which gives major originalities to the current study.

3. The operative time, change in haematocrit, presence of urinary leak, transfusion

requirement, _____ requirement, hospital stay and return to normal activity were analysed, as were complications, success rate and stent-related morbidity.

Answer: _____

Group 2

1. The present _____ is to make a percutaneous renal operation an outpatient procedure, which would be more palatable to patients and more cost-effective, without compromising safety.

2. Cardiovascular disease has become the number one eradicator of human life and substantial health _____ around the world.

3. Unfortunately, determining which patients with pulmonary infiltrates and impaired oxygenation will progress to ARDS remains a clinical _____.

Answer: _____

Group 3

1. Detection of these nascent stones could enable clinical intervention, such as a change of diet or addition of a _____, to prevent further stone growth.

2. All demographic, clinical, type of AF (paroxysmal, persistent and long lasting, permanent), laboratory and echocardiographic (including transoesophageal echocardiogram) data, as well as information on _____, were retrieved retrospectively from medical records.

3. The patients in the medication group had experienced more gouty attacks before starting _____ and had longer duration of gouty arthritis than patients in the no-medication group.

Answer: _____

Group 4

1. According to the present findings, the process of integration and reconstitution of self seems to _____ during pregnancy.

2. However, in progressive, predictive disease models of CP, a distinction between a RAP phase and onset of established CP is appropriate because it allows organization of risk and protective factors that may _____ or retard the expected rate of progression from RAP to early CP or established CP.

3. The implication of NGS data is that emerging pathogens will be members of genetic groups that have already been identified, and thus that comparison of an emerging disease X pathogen with known genetically related organisms would _____ vaccine development.

Answer: _____

| consistency | hospice | palliative | prolonged |

Group 5

1. Causes of death were assessed by additional review of inpatient, nursing home or _____ records, physician questionnaires and by interviews with next-of-kin.

2. All deaths that occurred under _____, nursing home care or in subjects with life-threatening non-cardiac comorbidities were not considered SCD.

3. She tolerated 2 cycles of treatment complicated by diarrhea, fatigue, and rash with stable disease as best response before experiencing clinical progression with recurrent right pleural effusion requiring an indwelling pleural drainage catheter. She was transitioned to home _____. Her survival was 11 months.

Answer: _____

Group 6

1. Systemic chemotherapy is also the primary _____ treatment of colorectal cancer metastases, as seen in cases of advanced hepatic involvement and in cases of liver metastasis recurrence following surgical resection.

2. Although TACE is primarily used in _____ situations, this technique can also be performed in a neoadjuvant intend.

3. Therefore, the novel concept of ASF therapy in combination with hormone ablation therapy is of clinical significance and merits further testing as a _____ approach regarding its efficacy, efficiency and its effect on quality of life, in comparison to salvage chemotherapy, in a randomized controlled trial setting for patients early in the progression to stage D3.

Answer: _____

Group 7

1. However, few circulating miRNAs so far have been reported as markers of CRC prognosis with limited _____ across different studies.

2. To maximize _____ and repeatability of data, five replications from five consecutive sections were obtained for lesion-to-background CNR measurements.

3. The result of ultra sound showed high _____ with CT and the progression of pneumonia.

Answer: _____

Group 8

1. In addition, TRPM7 suppression eliminated the need for the anti-excitotoxic cocktail to rescue anoxic neurons and permitted the survival of neurons previously destined to die from _____ anoxia.

2. Sacral osteoporotic fractures are frequent especially in elderly women and are a cause of _____ disability and immobilization, thereby worsening osteoporosis.

3. However, _____ survival may be achieved in selected patients; among the nine patients who survived at least 5 years, five survived longer than 10 years (131,146, 148,178, and 191 months).

Answer: _____

III. Cloze

Fill in each of the following blanks with the most appropriate word from each of the four choices given.

The development by the second half of the twentieth century of new technologies and effective specific treatments for disease still left much suffering __1__ . As Professor Patrick Wall wrote in 1986, "Symptoms were placed on one side and therapy directed at [them] was denigrated." __2__ the same vein, when Aneurin Bevan introduced the National Health Service Bill to Parliament, he stated that he would "rather be kept __3__ in the efficient if cold altruism of a large hospital than expire in a gush of sympathy in a small one".

But what if no cure was possible and the end of life was inevitable? Referring particularly __4__ the hospice movement, Wall added that "the old methods of care and caring had to be rediscovered and the best of modern medicine had to be turned to the task of new study and therapy specifically directed at pain". Care, __5__ with an increasingly sound evidence base, was by then underpinned by the concept of "total pain" defined in 1964 __6__ including not only physical symptoms but also mental distress and social or spiritual problems. This approach met ready audiences among nursing and medical students during lectures or in articles, __7__ social workers and more gradually among senior members of the medical profession.

During the 1950s three important surveys of end-of-life care were undertaken. In 1952 a report based on the observations of district nurses throughout the UK of some 7,050 cases, published by the Marie Curie Memorial Foundation, __8__ appalling conditions of suffering and deprivation among many patients __9__ cancer at home. By 1960, Glyn Hughes had conducted a __10__ survey for the Gulbenkian Foundation. This included widespread consultations, 300 site visits and contacts with 600 family doctors. Conditions in charitable homes were judged seriously __11__ , with __12__ in financial support and staffing, and a large proportion of the nursing homes visited were deemed "quite unsuited—and in some cases __13__ actual neglect when measured by standards that can reasonably be expected", Hughes noted, "a serious gap in the

National Health Service with an unanswered question of where and ___14___ the elderly terminally ill would be cared for." Finally, a unique detailed study of the physical and mental distress of the dying was published by John Hinton in 1963. His observations from the wards of a London teaching hospital showed that much suffering remained ___15___ and also how most patients were well aware of their prognosis despite the lack of information normally given at that time.

1. A. address   B. addressing   C. unaddress   D. unaddressed
2. A. At   B. On   C. In   D. By
3. A. alive   B. live   C. living   D. lively
4. A. with   B. to   C. by   D. between
5. A. to match   B. matching   C. match   D. matched
6. A. to   B. as   C. for   D. by
7. A. as well   B. as well as   C. might as well   D. as the same as
8. A. revealed   B. revealing   C. veiled   D. veiling
9. A. died of   B. dying of   C. died from   D. dying from
10. A. nation   B. national   C. nationwide   D. national
11. A. enough   B. adequate   C. sufficient   D. inadequate
12. A. deficiencies B. lack   C. efficiency   D. inefficiencies
13. A. amount in   B. amounting in   C. amount to   D. amounting to
14. A. for whom   B. by whom   C. in whom   D. to whom
15. A. rested   B. untested   C. unrelieved   D. relieved

IV. Discussion and Presentation

Answer the following questions on the basis of your reading.

1. As a (would-be) doctor, how much do you know about hospice and palliative care in China? What implications can we get from the reading?

2. Until today, there's a lack of a complete set of textbooks on hospice and palliative care in China's medical education. Is it appropriate to make uncritical use of textbooks published by foreign publishers?

3. As for the medication availability, pain relief medication in large hospitals and specialized hospitals are easily available. But there's still limited medication in many areas in China. What's your understanding of the situation?

V. Translation

Ttranslate the following sentences into English.

1. 有些人将死亡视为禁忌,认为在临终病人面前谈论死亡会带来厄运,不利于病人的健康和康复。

   _____

2. 近年来,随着公众和专业人士愈加深刻地认识到对临终患者的临床护理不足,以及对治疗不充分或过度治疗带来的情感、伦理和经济成本的认识不断加深,临终关怀和姑息治疗这一新兴领域经历了巨大的发展。

   _____

3. 缺乏受过专业培训的医护人员和管理人员是阻碍中国姑息治疗服务发展的另一个因素。

   _____

4. 姑息治疗是为了缓解癌症或其他危及生命的疾病引起的症状,而不是治愈疾病。

   _____

5. 在本科、研究生和继续教育中,临终关怀教育的不足反映了一种医学文化,这种文化将死亡定义为失败,忽视了对临终病人的护理是职业成就和个人价值体现的来源之一。

   _____

VI. Further Readings

1. Correspondence：Current Awareness of Palliative Care in China
2. Editorial：Palliative Care in China—Current Status and Future Directions
3. The Influence of Culture on End-of-Life Decision Making

Part II Academic Development

I. Transalting Medical Texts

Read the following sample abstract and put the underlined part into English.

【摘要】**目的**：系统评价居家安宁疗护对晚期癌症患者生活质量和情绪的影响，为相关研究提供循证依据。**方法**：计算机检索中国知网、万方数据库、维普数据库、中国生物医学文献数据库、CINAHL、CENTRAL、PubMed、Web of Science、Embase 中关于居家安宁疗护对晚期癌症患者的随机对照试验，并追踪参考文献，检索时限为建库至 2020 年 11 月 13 日。由 2 名研究者独立筛选文献并交叉核对纳入文献质量，按照 Cochrane 评价手册 5.1.0 的质量评价方法评价纳入文献质量。采用 RevMan 5.3 软件进行 Meta 分析。**结果**：共纳入 10 篇文献，包括 1 720 例晚期癌症患者。Meta 分析结果显示，居家安宁疗护可以改善晚期癌症患者的生活质量[SMD = 0.41, 95%CI(0.30, 0.51), Z = 7.44, P<0.001]，减轻抑郁情绪[SMD = −0.29, 95%CI(−0.45, −0.14), Z = 3.68, P<0.001]，尚不能认为居家安宁疗护能够减轻晚期癌症患者的焦虑情绪[SMD = −0.15, 95%CI(−2.12, 1.82), Z = 0.15, P = 0.880]。**结论**：居家安宁疗护能够提高晚期癌症患者的生活质量，减轻患者的抑郁情绪，暂未发现能够减轻患者的焦虑情绪，需高质量、大样本研究进一步探讨居家安宁疗护对患者的影响。[①]

> ### Translation & Writing Skills：Punctuations

Punctuations，seemingly to be trival matters though，play a very important role in expressing ideas. They improve sentence cadence and clarity and thus make reading easier. Take a look at the fowllowing two examples. The different placement of commas can actually result in completely different meanings.

> **Example 1**：The physician thought the patient looked gravely ill.

> **Example 2**：The physician，thought the patient，looked gravely ill.

In the above examples，the presence or absence of commas changes who seemed ill.

In translation，we must be careful with punctuations not only in their proper usages but also be fully aware of the differences between Chinese and English. Here are 5 of the most common punctuation marks which are different in Chinese compared to English

---

① 选自《中华护理杂志》2021 年第 8 期，1249 − 1255 页。作者：苏孟宇，王真，张玉玺，王婷，吴金凤。

and frequently misused in students' translations.

Punctuation Mark in Chinese	English Name	Chinese Name	May Appear in English as
。	Full Stop	句号	.
、	Enumeration comma	顿号	,
《 》	Title mark	书名号	italic or capitalized
……	Ellipsis	省略号	. . .
·	Middle dot	间隔号	space

Example 3：

混配农药中毒的其他危险因素还有：工间吸烟或进食、喷雾器发生故障或滴漏、施药后不能尽快清洗全身、个人防护不严密和长时间施药等。

Other risk factors for pesticide poisoning with mixed preparation were smoking or taking food during spraying，leaking or breakdown of sprayers，without washing their body as soon as possible after spraying，poor personal protection and spraying for a long time.

Example 4：

党中央、国务院高度重视人民健康，2016 年发布《"健康中国 2030"规划纲要》，提出了健康中国建设的目标和任务。

The CPC Central Committee and the State Council attach great importance to the people's health. In 2016，the State Council issued the *"Healthy China 2030" Planning Outline*，which put forward the goals and tasks of building a healthy China.

II. Writing Medical Papers in English

General Considerations for Results Section
By Zahra Bahadoran，et al.

The Results section is the heart of the paper，around which the other sections are organized. The function of the Results section is to present the main results of experiments described in the Materials and Methods section and to present the supporting data in the form of text，tables，and figures. This section should answer the basic question："What did the authors find in research?" By providing the results，authors try to elucidate the research data，making it to the point and meaningful.

Results and Data

This section includes both results and data that are presented in text, tables, and figures. Providing results but no data vs data but no results should be avoided. However, we need to bear in mind that data and results are not the same. Results are general statements in the main text that summarize or explain what the data (facts and numbers) show; in other words, results are text descriptions of what is important about data and give meaning to the data. When reporting data or results, make sure that they are logical. See Table 1 for more differences between results and data.

Table 1   Differences Between Results and Data

Data	Results
The facts (often numbers) obtained from experiments or observations.	The meaning and interpretation of data.
Can be presented as raw (e.g. concentration of a measured variable), summarized (e.g. mean and SD), or transformed (e.g. percentage).	Are expressed as statements that explain or summarize what the data show.
Can rarely stand alone.	May have a direction (e.g. decrease, increase) or magnitude, e.g. 2-fold, 10% increased.
	May contain statistical significance, e.g. P value.
E. g. Mean (SD) fasting blood glucose was 180(20) mg/dL in patients with type 2 diabetes. Mean fasting blood glucose was 95 (5) mg/dL in non-diabetic subjects.	E. g. mean fasting blood glucose was significantly higher in patients with type 2 diabetes than in non-diabetic subjects [180(20) vs 95(5) mg/dL, $P = 0.010$]*.

* The text presented in square brackets is data and the remainder is a result.

Length and Paragraphing

To see the forest for the tree, the Results section should be as brief and uncluttered as possible, which can be accomplished by having a well-organized Materials and Methods section and avoiding unnecessary repetition; for example, similar results for several variables can be reported together. The Results section of an original manuscript usually includes 2-3 pages ($\sim$ 1,000 words) with a 1.5 line spacing, font size 11 (including tables and figures), and 4-9 paragraphs (each 130 words) on average; a paragraph should be devoted to one or more closely related figures.

Presenting additional results/data as supplementary materials is a suggestion for keeping the Results section brief. In addition to save the text space, supplementary materials improve the presentation and facilitate communications among scientists. According to Springer, supplementary materials can be used for presenting data that are not needed to support the major conclusions but are still interesting. However, keep in mind that the unregulated use of supplementary materials is harmful to science. Supplementary materials should be referred to at the appropriate points in the main text.

Tense

For referring to results obtained in hypothesis testing studies, using past tenses is recommended; non-textual elements should be referred using present tenses, e. g. "as seen in Table 1..." or "Table 1 shows..." in descriptive studies, results are reported in the present tense.

Word Choice

Although adverbs/adjectives are commonly used to highlight the importance of results, it is recommended altogether avoiding the use of such qualitative/emotive words in the Results section. Some believe that qualitative words should not be used because they may imply an interpretation of findings. In biomedical publications, the terms "significant, significance, and significantly" (followed by P values) are used to show statistical relationships and should not be used for other purposes for which, other terms such as substantial, considerable, or noteworthy can be used. See Box 3 for appropriate word choice for the Results section.

Table 2   Some Do's and Don'ts for Word Choice in a Results Section

Do's
Use straightforward verbs for stating results, e. g. *show*, *indicate*, *demonstrate*, *highlight*, *identify*, *detect*, *observe*, *find*, and *confirm*.
Use "significant" or "significantly" just for statistical significance.
Be careful about using negative sentences:
Instead of using double negatives, be straightforward and use positive terms.
Make the sentence clear by omitting negative words or negative sentence constructions, e. g. "There was no significant interaction..." instead of "We did not find a statistical interaction...."

Don'ts
Do not use "reveal" to state the results because it is a funny word that suggests something was found perhaps by magic.
Do not use emotive words to describe the significance of the results, e. g. *interestingly*, *unfortunately*, *curiously*, *remarkably*, *inexplicably*, *importantly*, *crucially*, and *critically*.
Do not use the word "level" instead of "concentration".

In the Results section, to make a comparison between the results, i. e. stating the similarity/equivalence or difference/non-equivalence, using appropriate signals is recommended. To show a similarity, a signal to the reader may be used such as "like" "alike" "similar to" and "the same as"; to show differences, the following signals can be used: "but" "while" "however" "in contrast" "more likely than", and "less likely than".

Reporting Numbers

Numbers play an important role in scientific communication and there are some golden rules for reporting numbers in a scientific paper. Significant figures (significant digits) should reflect the degree of precision of the original measurement. The number of digits reported for a quantity should be consistent with scientific relevance; for example, a resolution to 0.001 units is necessary for pH but a resolution of <1 mmHg is unimportant for blood pressure. Avoid using "about" or "approximately" to qualify a measurement or calculation. The use of percentage for sample sizes of <20 and decimal for sample sizes of <100 is not recommended.

The numbers should be spelled out at the beginning of a sentence or when they are less than 10, e.g. twelve students improved... In a sentence, the authors should be consistent where they use numbers as numerals or spelled-out. Before a unit of a measure, time, dates, and points, numbers should be used as numerals, e.g. 12 cm, 1 h 34 min, at 12:30 A.M., and on a 7-point scale.

A space between the numeral and the unit should be considered, except in the case of %. Because the terms "billion" "trillion", and "quadrillion" imply different numbers in Europe and the USA, they should not be used. To express ranges in text, the terms "to" or "through" are preferred to dashes; in tables, the use of dashes or hyphens is recommended.

Table 3　Do's and Don'ts of Writing a Results Section

Do's
Present demographics or simple descriptive statistics first.
Describe results from the most to the least important and from the primary outcomes to the secondary outcomes.
Organize the Results section using separate headings as in Methods section or by categories.
Make up the Results section using a combination of text, tables, and figures.
Quantify results using appropriate indicators of centrality, probability, and statistical significance values.
Match each result by its corresponding assessment/measurement method.
Be focused on results related to the research hypothesis/question.
Provide units according to the journal style and in a constant manner throughout the text.

续　表

Don'ts
Report all analyses including those unrelated to the main study hypothesis/question.
Compare the study results with those of previous reports.
Discuss and interpret the results.
Restate similar results in both textual and non-textual elements.
Present raw data.
Present data lacking units of measurements.
Present crowded and confusing tables or figures.

The Results section of a biomedical manuscript should clearly present findings of the study using an effective combination of results and data. Some do's and don'ts of writing the Results section are provided in Table 3. Authors should try to find the best format using a dynamic interplay between text and figures/tables. Results can be organized in different ways including chronological order or most to least important; however, results should be presented in a manner that makes sense.

Unit 7

Gene Editing and Human Dignity

📖 **Lead-in** What Is Gene Editing?

Task 1 *Watch the video and answer the following questions, and then exchange your answers with your classmates.*

1. What is gene editing according to the video?

_____

_____

2. Can you enumerate any human characteristics that can be influenced by DNA?

_____

_____

3. What could be the potential benefits and possible negatives of gene editing?

_____

_____

Task 2 *Watch the video again and fill the following gaps. Make sure the word (s) you fill in is (are) both grammatically and semantically acceptable.*

Genes are sections of the long DNA molecules (1) _____ inside each cell of every living thing from (2) _____ and insects to plants and animals including humans.

DNA is inherited from our parents. We have a (3) _____ of two sets of genes, one from each parent brought together to produce a new set of (4) _____

_____ and (5) _____ .

　　Gene editing is already (6) _____ , but at this early stage of such a powerful technology, it's crucial that we (7) _____ against the possible negatives.

Part I　Intensive Reading

Human Dignity and Gene Editing

By Iñigo de Miguel Beriain

1　The emergence of gene editing technology—particularly CRISPR-Cas9—and the first experiments to modify the genome of human embryos have given rise to an intense ethical debate. Such an in-depth discussion of the potential ethical, societal and medical implications is indeed highly relevant as modifications of the germline would not only affect individual patients or humans but the human species as a whole. In fact, the debate began even before the availability of the CRISPS/Cas system when the first gene therapies were developed to cure a few select pathologies. Time has not brought any general agreement, and a universal consensus on whether or not to allow human germline editing is still remote.

2　While some commentators call for a total ban on any form of gene editing that affects the human germline, others advocate for a moratorium until the risks have been sufficiently addressed and resolved. Some even claim that germline editing should be considered a moral imperative to improve the human species. Similar disagreements exist about the ends to which these techniques should be applied. Some consider that only therapeutic purposes are acceptable; others support their use for human enhancement, a view that many bioethicists and most international declarations and conventions consider as a form of eugenics.

3　A clear definition of human dignity remains elusive, because the concept of dignity is, in itself, extremely problematic to the extent that some people consider that it should be completely omitted from bioethics. For the sake of the argument that human dignity should not be an obstacle to genome editing, it is not necessary to delve too deep into this controversy. It is enough to summarize that those who believe in the importance of human dignity and its relation to the human genome generally share three main ideas.

4　The first is that dignity—which is linked to the concept of autonomy—is an intrinsic and non-negotiable value shared by all human beings, simply by virtue of belonging to the human species. This idea has deep roots in our collective imagination. Second, advocates of the idea of human dignity believe that since every human being has the same intrinsic moral value, every person should be treated as though he or she was an end in his or herself and not a mere means. Third, there is a broad tendency in bioethics to directly link the notion of human dignity to the human genome. Since it is the genome that determines who belongs to the human species and since being part of the human species confers dignity, it seems reasonable to link human dignity to the human genome.

5 As previously noted, various authors believe that human dignity is intrinsically linked to the human genome. The question then is as follows: What are the normative implications of this belief? The general opinion among opponents of germline editing is that since our dignity is embedded in our genome, we must refrain from altering. If one believes that our dignity can only remain undiminished if the human genome remains unchanged, we cannot tolerate any new mutation in the human genome—regardless of whether it is produced by human action or naturally. A major fallacy of arguments based on preserving the human genome is ignoring the fact that the human genome is not a fixed entity, an immutable biological substrate, but subject to mutations like any other genome: otherwise, evolution would come to a halt. Even more so, if we claim that respect for human dignity means preserving the human genome in its current state, the logical conclusion would be not only to renounce sexual reproduction in favor of cloning—as it generates mutations—but even to use gene editing to remove any natural, random mutations because it might violate human dignity and autonomy.

6 Those who argue for the need to preserve the human genome draw a subtle distinction between direct actions that deliberately introduce changes such as gene therapy or therapeutic gene editing and actions that introduce mutations indirectly as a side effect, such as radio- or chemotherapy that carry a risk of generating mutations of germline cells. Indeed, a sizeable number of ethicists and some of our main regulatory instruments argue that direct actions to change the human genome are morally reprehensible and must therefore be illegal. However, interventions that tolerate such changes may be morally acceptable for the sake of defending a greater good. If we accept that our dignity is linked to the human genome and that any change in the latter affects the former, it is not clear why the type of action—direct or indirect—and not its result should be relevant. Is it really pivotal whether the genome has been altered directly or as an inevitable consequence of the action? If human dignity is compromised by the alteration of the human genome, then it clearly does not make a difference. But

if so, why should we accept one type of alteration and reject the other?

7 Therefore, if we believe that any change in the genome caused by human action is a breach of human dignity, we must refrain from any kind of action that could lead to this consequence whether directly or indirectly even if this means abolishing radio or chemotherapy. The fact that this appeal does not arise often is a clear inconsistency that can be justified only on pragmatic grounds. But this justification is an unacceptable trick when human dignity is at stake. Last but not least, a consciously caused alteration of the human genome is much closer to the idea of autonomy than is random change brought about by chemotherapy. Again, inconsistencies in the more conservative discourse appear to give a poor answer to this question. Therefore, if we are to accept actions that alter the human genome, even if indirectly, then we have plenty of reasons to consider that those intended to directly produce such a result should also be considered morally acceptable on the basis of human dignity.

8 There is a big difference between changing the genome of a human being and changing the human genome. This is not dependent on whether it is the genome of one or several human beings, or whether the change occurs in the somatic or germinal line. It depends on the type of alteration. If the final result of the intervention for instance—replacing a mutated gene to restore its original function—does not introduce any novelty into the human gene pool, then it is inaccurate to speak of an alteration in the human genome.

9 Imagine, for example, a human embryo with mutations of the Huntington gene that will inevitably lead to Huntington's disease if the embryo grows into a human being. If we edit its germline to replace the gene with a normal variant, we will modify the embryo's genome but not the human genome. The ultimate result of the intervention—a human being with a genome that does not show the specific pathological variant that triggers Huntington's disease—will not introduce any novelty into the human gene pool. Therefore, any appeal not to carry out such intervention on the basis of the defense of the human genome and, hence, human dignity, would be manifestly illogical.

10 The overall conclusion is that there are no good reasons to justify a general ban on genetic editing of the human germline on the basis of human dignity. On the contrary, it is precisely this factor that should prompt us to use genome editing in the interests of the individual human being. Given the logical fallacies, it seems about time to give up on a notion of human dignity and autonomy that is closely linked to the human genome and consider each of these separately when discussing the ethical implications of human genome and germline editing.

Words and Expressions

CRISPR — clustered regularly interspaced short palindromic repeats

embryo /ˈembriəʊ/ *n.* — an unborn animal or human being in the very early stages of development

modification /ˌmɒdɪfɪˈkeɪʃn/ *n.* — the act of making something different (as e. g. the size of a garment)

consensus /kənˈsensəs/ *n.* — general agreement among a group of people

advocate /ˈædvəkeɪt/ *n.* — a person who pleads for a cause or propounds an idea

moratorium /ˌmɔːrəˈtɔːriəm/ *n.* — the act of stopping of a particular activity or process for a fixed period of time

eugenics /juːˈdʒenɪks/ *n.* — the study of methods to improve human race by carefully selecting parents who will produce the healthiest children

elusive /ɪˈluːsɪv/ *adj.* — difficult to find, describe, remember, or achieve

intrinsic /ɪnˈtrɪnsɪk/ *adj.* — belonging to a thing by its very nature

normative /ˈnɔːmətɪv/ *adj.* — pertaining to giving directives or rules

opponent /əˈpəʊnənt/ *n.* — someone who offers opposition

renounce /rɪˈnaʊns/ *v.* — to turn away from; to give up

substrate /ˈsʌbstreɪt/ *n.* — a surface on which an organism grows or is attached

imperative /ɪmˈperətɪv/ *n.* — something which is extremely important and must be done

refrain /rɪˈfreɪn/ *v.* — to resist doing something

undiminished /ˌʌndɪˈmɪnɪʃt/ *adj.* — not reduced or lessened

mutation /mjuːˈteɪʃn/ *n.* — any alteration in the inherited nucleic acid sequence of the genotype of an organism

fallacy /ˈfæləsi/ *n.* — a misconception resulting from incorrect reasoning

reprehensible /ˌreprɪˈhensəbl/ *adj*.   deserving censure or condemnation

pivotal /ˈpɪvətl/ *adj*.   being of crucial importance

pragmatic /præɡˈmætɪk/ *adj*.   dealing with things sensibly and realistically in a way that is based on practical rather than theoretical conside- rations

variant /ˈveəriənt/ *n*.   a group of organisms within a species that differ in trivial ways from similar groups

intervention /ˌɪntəˈvenʃn/ *n*.   action taken to improve a situation, especially a medical disorder

conservative /kənˈsɜːvətɪv/ *adj*.   resistant to change

somatic /səʊˈmætɪk/ *adj*.   relating to the body

I. Reading Comprehension

Choose the best answer to each of the following questions.

1. Which statement is true according to the author's point of view on gene editing?
    A. Using human dignity as an argument against modifying the human genome and germline is a logical fallacy.
    B. Human dignity is intrinsically linked to the human genome that we must refrain from altering it.
    C. Respect for human dignity should actually support arguments to veto any alterations of human genome.
    D. Germline modification would threaten human dignity as human genome is the physical representation of it.

2. Which one of the ideas below is NOT generally shared by people who believe in the importance of human dignity and its relation to the human genome?
    A. All human beings are born free and equal in dignity and rights.
    B. We can instrumentalize human beings.
    C. Trafficking in human beings constitutes an offence to the dignity of human being.
    D. In a symbolic sense, human genome is the heritage of humanity.

3. The author mentions "sexual reproduction" and "cloning" to _____ .
    A. justify that cloning is a better way to preserve human genome
    B. emphasize that sexual reproduction would generate mutations
    C. argue that human genome is naturally mutable

D. remind us that the human dignity remains unchanged only if human genome remains unchanged

4. What is the purpose of explaining mutations of the Huntington gene?

A. Such interventions could constitute an indirect threat to human dignity.

B. Such interventions can cure Huntington's disease in embryo or in a human being.

C. Such interventions do not change human gene.

D. Such interventions can improve human species.

5. What is the author's opinion on the distinction between direct and indirect actions to change human genome?

A. Both of them compromise human dignity by altering the human genome.

B. They don't make a difference and should be considered morally acceptable.

C. Only indirect actions such as radio or chemotherapy should be justified.

D. Direct alterations with good intentions may be acceptable.

II. Vocabulary

Task 1 *Fill in the blanks of the following sentences with the words or expressions given in the box below. Change the forms where necessary.*

embryo	modification	consensus	variant	pragmatic
refrain	fallacy	opponent	pivotal	renounce
elusive	advocate	imperative	mutation	moratorium

1. The woman who exhibited the _____ was immunocompromised as she had previously been treated for non-Hodgkin's lymphoma.

2. She considers it a moral _____ to help people in need.

3. The _____ of their ideas about medicine soon became apparent.

4. Since I am not very good at math, earning an "A" in geometry is an _____ goal for me.

5. The idea is that the male mosquitoes—made sterile through bacteria, gene _____ or X-ray—will mate with the females and produce non-viable eggs, driving down the population.

6. There is no _____ on how many people must be vaccinated to stop the pandemic, but experts agree that 50% is nowhere close.

7. A new _____ of the disease has appeared.

8. Her advice to those in entry-level accounting and finance positions is to be _____

in acquiring new skills such as technology and data science, as well as understanding general business principles like leadership and management.

9. Many of his former supporters have _____ him.

10. The director of the blood bank called for a _____ in donations until the surplus could be used up.

11. If an _____ inherits a faulty copy of a gene from one parent, the copy from the other parent can compensate.

12. Ms. Hart was familiar with local medical-review policies from her work as a patient _____.

13. Coaches can plan _____ specific strategies and tactical changes in games based on insights from hard data.

14. The consultants issued a company-wide memorandum requesting that employees _____ from using abusive language.

15. Among the many vitamins and omega fatty acids in this body-smoother, vitamin B3 plays a _____ role.

Task 2 *Under each of the following boxes there are several groups of sentences. In each sentence a common word or expression is missing. Find it out from the corresponding box according to the meaning and structure of the sentences. The forms of the words and expressions may change in the sentences.*

intervention   conservative   intrinsic   somatic

Group 1

1. Case 1 reveals a more _____ approach, where single agent vinorelbine was offered as first-line, reflecting the standard of care at the time, but the patient ultimately declined chemotherapy.

2. It deals with indications and results of 60 consecutive patients with moderate to severe stenosis, neurological symptoms and failure of _____ treatment.

3. In conjunction with other _____ measures to treat pain in knee OA, intra-articular corticosteroid injections (IACI) are commonly used in accordance with published guidance.

Group 2

1. Patients with history of percutaneous coronary _____, arteriovenous graft, familial hypercholesterolemia and congenital defects of the heart valves were excluded.

2. They could show similar findings between _____ and placebo groups in the incidence of ventricular arrhythmia and episodes of ST-segment depression, length of QTc, and systolic and diastolic echocardiographic measures as well as 1-year AEs including death, recurrent acute coronary syndrome, or need to repeating revascularization.

3. An asymptomatic dry eye from a positive test only is of uncertain clinical importance and does not warrant therapeutic _____.

Group 3

1. The presence of these regulatory cells in cancer patients could be important in inducing T-cell suppression, thus allowing tumor growth. In addition, the T cells themselves may have _____ defects.

2. Results across many cancer cell types have reported activation of the _____ apoptotic pathway following DATS treatment.

3. This implies that the buildup of DNA damage over time is not solely responsible for hematopoietic dysfunction and that FA cells possess additional _____ pathophysiologic properties.

Group 4

1. The oncogenic potential of HER2/neu in human neoplasms has been shown to be due to gene amplification and overexpression of the gene product and is not associated with a _____ mutation.

2. Clearly, an elevated mutation rate may make the _____ malignant evolution faster, but is not necessary for malignancies to occur.

3. _____ pain accompanies arthritis, bone or spine metastases, low back pain, and orthopaedic procedures.

manifest	compromise	confer	subtle

Group 5

1. Involvement of other subsets, such as regulatory T cells and macrophages, has been investigated, showing that they can _____ either good or poor prognosis depending on context.

2. Alternatively, these proteins may _____ resistance through hydrophobic interactions with structured molecules.

3. Because much of the pathophysiology associated with I/R injury is centred on microvascular disruption, CO generation is likely to _____ significant benefits.

Group 6

1. Patients with diffuse interstitial lung disease must cautiously decide whether to undergo a lobectomy, which may _____ lung function after surgery.

2. These mismatches can _____ the effectiveness of miRNA activity.

3. Although concern has been expressed that a lower diastolic BP together with reduced diastolic flow in the descending aorta may significantly _____ flow to the kidneys, liver and gut.

Group 7

1. Nonsecretory myeloma is defined by the absence of serum or urinary (or both) monoclonal immunoglobulins in patients who otherwise _____ features typically found in multiple myeloma.

2. Adverse drug reactions will almost always _____ within 24 hours.

3. We establish the inadequacy of commercially available colorectal cancer (CRC) lines to _____ chemotherapy resistance, an observation clearly demonstrated in our patient derived cancer-initiating cells (CICs).

Group 8

1. Possible mechanisms of cytochrome c release data from our lab and from others clearly show that cytochrome c release can happen in a very _____ way leaving much of mitochondrial structure and function intact.

2. Additionally, the ability of wave-intensity analysis to recognize the _____ differences in biventricular pacing regimens has been highlighted.

3. Recent findings show that even low cadmium burdens may cause _____ renal effects on the proximal tubule in children.

III. Cloze

Fill in each of the following blanks with the most appropriate word from each of the four choices given.

Genome editing, enabled by recent scientific advances, can generate targeted insertions and deletions in DNA and may even offer enough precision to modify a single base pair within the genome of an organism. Basic science research with genome editing is now ___1___ in laboratories globally. Human genome editing is also advancing rapidly, with clinical trials now ___2___ for prevention and treatment of various human diseases. These trials, which are currently in early stages, involve somatic (non reproductive) cells, and thus are not ___3___ to introduce genetic changes that will be ___4___ to offspring or the germline (reproductive) cells.

While genome editing holds great ___5___ to help improve human lives，the technology raises profound safety，ethical，legal，and social concerns. Safety concerns for genome editing include the risk of unintended or unforeseen ___6___ off-target effects （edits in the wrong place） unwanted on-target modifications （imprecise edits），and mosaicism （when only some cells carry the edits），and abnormal immunological responses. Ethical issues regarding genome editing include concerns that editing may be used for non-therapeutic and ___7___ purposes rather than for therapeutic purposes，i. e. improving health or curing disease. There are also concerns that germline modifications could create classes of individuals defined by the quality of their engineered genome，possibly enabling eugenics，which could ___8___ social inequalities or be used coercively. Legal issues include providing ___9___ for risk management and assignment of duties and ___10___，particularly when modifications can be passed to subsequent generations. There are also risks，both legal and ethical，involved in the proliferation of ___11___ direct-to-consumer CRISPR kits that allow individuals to undertake gene editing independently in a home setting. At a social level，debates ___12___ around the concerns that access to beneficial genome editing will be ___13___ （e. g. only the wealthy will have access） and will increase existing ___14___ in health and medical care.

Human genome-editing，like any other medical intervention，should be implemented according to appropriate evidence that is collected via well-conducted and ethically approved research studies. When ___15___ the use of germline cells for research purposes，germline editing should be permitted only within a separate ethical and legal framework，distinct from an ethical and legal framework applied to somatic genome editing.

1. A. underlying   B. undertaking   C. underway   D. underline

2. A. in question   B. in progress   C. in use   D. adequacy

3. A. desired   B. interested   C. participated D. anticipated

4. A. carry off   B. pass off   C. pass on   D. carry on

5. A. possibilities   B. hopes   C. significance D. potentials

6. A. pleiotropic   B. inotropic   C. carry   D. perform

7. A. selection   B. enhancement   C. development   D. advancement

8. A. impede   B. accelerate   C. exacerbate   D. degenerate

9. A. statement   B. clarity   C. instruction   D. clearance

10. A. credence   B. conformity   C. consistency   D. liabilities

11. A. unvalidated   B. unspecified

    C. unidentified   D. unrecognized

12. A. delve　　　　　　　　　B. involve

　　C. revolve　　　　　　　　D. revoke

13. A. inequitable　　　　　　　B. insufficient

　　C. impartial　　　　　　　　D. edit

14. A. distribution　　　　　　　B. allocation

　　C. disparities　　　　　　　D. dispute

15. A. manipulating　　　　　　　B. contemplating

　　C. implementing　　　　　　　D. speculating

IV. Discussion and Presentation

Answer the following questions on the basis of your reading.

1. What do you think of the broad tendency in bioethics to directly link the notion of human dignity to the human genome?

2. What is (are) potentially at stake with new gene-editing technologies?

3. Try to explore the possibilities and challenges of applying genome-editing techniques to better understand the scientific aspects of the human germline. And make recommendations on the ethnical considerations regarding the use of genetic technology in health care.

V. Translation

Translate the following sentences into English.

1. 大多数与基因组编辑相关的伦理讨论都围绕着人类种系展开,因为在种系中所做的编辑改变将遗传给后代。

　　_____

　　_____

2. 与许多新技术一样,人们担心基因组编辑会成为富人的独享权利,并且在医疗和介入治疗服务可及性方面导致已有的差异进一步加大。

　　_____

　　_____

3. 研究人员和生物伦理学家还担心由于种系治疗的风险未知,因此能否真正获得准父母们的知情同意还不得而知。

　　_____

　　_____

4. 基因编辑的大部分工作都是在医疗领域进行的,其中一些最激动人心的项目专注于"纠正"可能导致严重疾病的 DNA 突变。

5. 为预防疾病或改善健康而进行的基因编辑工作可分为两类。第一种是种系疗法,它可以引起生殖细胞(卵子和精子)的变化,从而引起后代遗传的变化。第二种是体细胞,它以非生殖细胞为靶向,有可能治愈或减缓疾病在目标生物体内的传播。

VI. Further Readings

1. Gene Editing and Ethics

2. Ethical Considerations Regarding the Use of Genetics in Health Care

3. Human Genome Editing：Recommendations

 Part II Academic Development

I. Translating Medical Texts

Read the following sample abstract and put the underlined part into English.

【摘要】人类胚胎基因编辑引发了全球生物学家、生命伦理学者、社会公众等激烈的伦理论争。反对者认为,人类胚胎基因编辑突破了不可逾越的伦理"红线",应当"全面禁止",理由主要有：改写人类进化方式;存在严重技术风险;违背后代自决权;导致人类社会新的不平等;损害人类的"基因完整性"与"人种完整性"。而支持者认为,人类胚胎基因编辑有利于探究生命奥秘和促进人类健康,具有科学及道德合理性,应当"全面开放"。面对这一巨大而深刻的伦理悖论,本文提出了"有限开放"的解悖路径,即实现人类胚胎基因编辑的差异性发展,使之"弃恶扬善",同时,构筑立体的人类胚胎基因编辑监管体系,为其伦理悖论的化解提供制度保障。①

> **Translation & Writing Skills：Hypotaxis vs. Parataxis Between English & Chinese**

There is a contrast between English and Chinese that is hypotaxis and parataxis. Hypotaxis is the grammatical arrangement of functionally similar but "unequal" constructs，i. e. certain constructs have more importance than others inside a sentence. Parataxis favors short，simple sentences，with the use of coordinating rather

---

① 选自《自然辩证法通讯》2018 年第 2 期,85-91 页。作者：陶应时,罗成翼。

than subordinating conjunctions. English features more of hypotaxis whereas Chinese of parataxis. To put it simple, we can use an analogy to show the difference between the two. English is like a tree whose branches are all intertwined, whereas Chinese is like a bamboo whose stems build upon one another.

Compare the following English and Chinese sentences to have a better understanding of hypotaxis and parataxis.

> **English:** The boy, *who* was crying as if his heart would break, said, *when* I spoke to him, *that* he was hungry *because* he had had no food for two days.
> **Chinese:** 男孩哭得很伤心，我问他怎么了，他说他太饿了，已经两天没吃东西了。

In the Chinese translation, the sentence spreads out part by part gradually just like a bamboo.

> 男孩哭得很伤心→我问他怎么了→他说他太饿了→已经两天没吃东西了。

However, the English sentence has a more complex structure.

> The boy←who was crying←as if his heart would break
> ↓
> said←when I spoke to him
> ↓
> that he was hungry←because he had had no food for two days

The trunk of the tree, that is, the main clause of the sentence, is "The boy said that he was hungry", and there are quite a few clauses in this sentence: "who was crying" is an attributive clause to modify "the boy", and "as if his heart would break" is an adverbial clause to modify the verb "cry", which indicates the manner. Moreover, "when I spoke to him" is an adverbial clause to modify the verb "said". which indicates the time. In addition, "because he had had no food for two days" is an adverbial clause to show the reason for "hungry". In both translation and writting practice, we need to be conscious of this distinction between English and Chinese.

Examples:

> **Example 1:** Luckily, *at this time* he caught a liver complaint, for the cure of *which* he returned to Europe, and *which* was the source of great comfort and amusement to him in his native country.
> 算他运气好，正在那时害了肝病，必须回到欧洲去医治，才算有机会在本国享福。

Example 2：The problem is, this ignores the fact *that* it is not so much the intervention itself as the focus and process of research *that* make it profoundly different from innovation.

问题本身在于其忽略了一个事实：干预在其中起的作用并不大，而是研究本身的重点和过程使其很大程度上与创新有很大区别。

Example 3：卵巢淋巴管与血管伴行至下腹部的腹主动脉处，最终注入到腹主动脉旁淋巴结。

Lymphatic drainage of the ovaries follows the ovarian vessels to the lower abdominal aorta, where they drain into the para-aortic nodes.

Example 4：尽管与患者的交流有多种风格，每一个医生都应该确立一种自己与患者交流最佳的方式，医生必须告诉患者，他们可以并且也乐意倾听，所有他们所得到的信息均将得到最大程度的保密。

Although there are many styles of interacting with patients, and each physician must develop and determine the best way that he or she can relate to patients, physicians must convey that they are able and willing to listen and that they receive the information with utmost confidentiality.

Example 5：中国将积极推动中医药走向世界，促进中医药等传统医学与现代科学技术的有机结合，探索医疗卫生保健的新模式，服务于世界人民的健康福祉，开创人类社会更加美好的未来，为世界文明发展作出更大贡献。

China will also actively introduce TCM to the rest of the world, and promote the integration of TCM and other traditional medicines with modern technology, so as to explore a new model of healthcare to improve the well-being of all people of the world, and make a full contribution to global progress and a brighter future for mankind.

II. Writing Medical Papers in English

How to Write a Thoughtful Discussion

The discussion needs to be just that—a discussion. It isn't enough to simply rehash your results; you need to situate your research in the context of previous studies, draw out the practical implications of your own research, address limitations, and suggest areas for future study. Only then will your paper be ready for submission to a journal and the peer-review process. So, what are the keys to success when writing a scientific discussion? We've pulled together a few do's and don'ts to keep in mind.

What to Do When Writing a Scientific Discussion

1. Do Summarize Your Results and Outline Their Interpretation in Light of the Published Literature

This is the first thing that you need to do when writing a scientific discussion section. Use the first paragraph to describe very briefly the conclusion from your results, and then explain what it means with respect to what is already known from previous studies. Try to highlight the practical implications of your findings, and ensure that you demonstrate your ability to think critically about your main findings.

Remember to emphasize how your results support or refute the current hypotheses in the field, if any. Try to offer alternative explanations of results. This is also a good place to address if your data conflict with what is established in the field. By addressing these conflicts, other researchers in your field will re-examine and rebuild hypotheses/ models to test.

Keep in mind that all results should be discussed, and all parts of the discussion should relate to your results; don't ignore any results and don't discuss anything that doesn't relate to the results obtained.

2. Do Explain the Importance of Your Results

Be sure to advocate for your findings and underline how your results significantly move the field forward. Remember to give your results their due and don't undermine them. Make sure you mention the most important finding first; this is what people will remember.

3. Do Acknowledge the Shortcomings of the Study

In this section, explicitly state any potential limitations that your hypothesis or experimental approach might have and the reasoning behind them. This will help the field to generate hypotheses and new approaches without facing the same challenges. No study is perfect, and the discussion becomes well-rounded when you emphasize not only the impact of the study but also where it may fall short.

4. Do Discuss Any Future Directions

Depending on which journal you are publishing in, you might have to provide a separate "future directions" section, rather than having it tied into the discussion. Nonetheless, you should think about the questions that your study might lead to while you are writing the discussion. Consider posing a few questions, preferably in the form of a hypothesis, to provide a launchpad for future research.

5. Do Decide Between the Active or Passive Voice

Lots of journals stipulate writing in the active voice, as it is more immediate and concise. And because the active voice is more personal, it also creates a better connection with the reader.

e. g. *We analyzed the samples*.

Sometimes, however, the passive voice will be more appropriate if you wish to foreground the research rather than the researcher.

e. g. *The samples were analyzed*.

The passive voice is widely used in scientific communication as it creates a kind of objective distance between the researcher and the research. But at the same time, it can come across as a bit dry and impersonal. The key to writing engaging scientific papers is to vary your choice of the active and passive voice to best suit the point you're trying to make.

Make sure you also check the preference of your target journal and follow their style guide. Use the active voice if the people performing an action are important, but opt for the passive voice if it is the action rather than those who performed it that is key.

6. Do Pick Your Tenses Carefully

Scientific papers generally switch tenses between different sections of the paper. In the discussion section, a good rule of thumb is to stick to the past tense for describing completed actions (e. g. to summarize your findings).

e. g. *We measured the volumes of X and Y*.

You should use the present tense to interpret your results or to discuss the significance of your research findings:

e. g. *This is significant because X and Y are* . . .

Use the future tense to outline any work that is still to be done:

e. g. *In a follow-up study, we will measure Z*.

What NOT To Do While Writing a Scientific Discussion

Now that we've outlined the important features of an authoritative discussion section, here are a few pointers about things to avoid.

7. Don't Reiterate Your Results

You can open the discussion with a sentence that contains a snapshot of the main conclusion, but make sure you stop right there! You've already written a separate "results" section, so you don't want to go into too much detail or repeat yourself by describing your results again. Rather, swiftly transition into what these results mean and explain their impact.

8. Don't Over-interpret Your Findings

I mentioned giving your results their proper due and underscoring their significance. But be careful not to extrapolate your results and interpret something that is beyond the scope of the study.

Keep in mind the difference between what your results suggest at a given point versus what more can be known from them. You can do this by asking more questions and applying other experimental approaches.

Importantly, you must draw conclusions commensurate with your results.

9. Don't Introduce a New Piece of Data

Don't make the discussion confusing by introducing any new results or research questions. Present all of your data in the results section.

10. Don't Use Too Much Jargon

Although readers in your field of expertise would probably understand any jargon, try to minimize its use to make your paper accessible to a broader audience and to enable a larger impact. If you need to use abbreviations, for example, make sure that they're defined on the first mention. Even if a technique or reagent is more commonly known by an abbreviation, provide the full term in brackets.

You're trying to share knowledge, so your discussion should be as easy to read as possible. Try and use plain English and bear in mind that English may not be the mother tongue of many of your readers, so it's probably a good idea to avoid lots of idioms.

If you can use a shorter word for something, make sure you use it. Good writing is clear, concise, and simple, and this applies to science writing too. So choose "use" rather than "utilize", or "ask" rather than "enquire", for example.

This has nothing to do with dumbing-down, and everything to do with clarity; there's nothing to be gained from trying to make your writing sound overly scholarly or inaccessible. Check out the resources of the Plain English Campaign at http://www.plainenglish.co.uk/for more help.

This also shows why gathering feedback on your writing and editing your work are such important steps in the process of writing scientific manuscripts. You need to check how your paper sounds to someone else; if something doesn't make sense to one of your readers, it probably needs to be rewritten. In a nutshell, remember that the primary goal of writing a scientific discussion is to accentuate your results. Therefore, take the time to ensure that it is well-rounded, succinct, and relevant. Do all that and your paper should sail through peer review!

Unit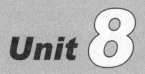

Language Problems for Non-native English Researchers

Lead-in : Why Did English Become the "Global Language"?

Task 1 *Watch the video and answer the following questions and then exchange your answers with your classmates.*

1. Can you explain what is "global language" in your own words?

_____

_____

2. What contributed to English's status of being the global language?

_____

_____

_____

Task 2 *Watch the video again and fill the following gaps. Make sure the word(s) you fill in is(are) both grammatically and semantically acceptable.*

A language becomes a global language because of (1) _____. It's nothing to do with the (2) _____. It's all to do with (3) _____ which means (4) _____.

English became international in the the 16th and 17th century because of (5) _____
_____ ; in the 18th century because of (6) _____ ; in the 19th century because of (7) _____ when America and Britain had (8) _____

134

_____ ; and then in the 20th century because (9) _____ .

Part I　Intensive Reading

English Is the Language of Science—That Isn't Always a Good Thing
By Ben Panko

1 Thirteen years ago, a deadly strain of avian flu known as H5N1 was tearing through Asia's bird populations. In January 2004, Chinese scientists reported that pigs too had become infected with the virus—an alarming development, since pigs are susceptible to human viruses and could potentially act as a "mixing vessel" that would allow the virus to jump to humans. "Urgent attention should be paid to the pandemic preparedness of these two sub-types of influenza," the scientists wrote in their study. Yet at the time, little attention was paid outside of China—because the study was published only in Chinese, in a Chinese journal of veterinary medicine.

2 It wasn't until August of that year that the World Health Organization and the United Nations learned of the study's results and rushed to have it translated. Those scientists and policy makers ran headlong into one of science's biggest unsolved dilemmas: language. A new study in the journal *PLOS Biology* sheds light on how widespread the gulf can be between English-language science and any-other-language science, and how that gap can lead to situations like the avian flu case, or worse.

3 "Native English speakers tend to assume that all important information is in English," says Tatsuya Amano, a zoology researcher at the University of Cambridge and lead author on this study. Amano, a native of Japan who has lived in Cambridge for five years, has encountered this bias in his own work as a zoologist; publishing in English was essential for him to further his career, he says. At the same time, he has seen studies that have been overlooked by global reviews, presumably because they were only published in Japanese. Yet particularly when it comes to work about biodiversity and conservation, Amano says, much of the most important data is collected and published by researchers in the countries where exotic or endangered species live—not just the United States or England. This can lead to oversights of important statistics or critical breakthroughs by international organizations, or even scientists unnecessarily duplicating research that has already been done. Speaking for himself and his collaborators, he says: "We think ignoring non-English papers can cause biases in your understanding." His study offers concrete examples of the consequences of science's English bias. For instance, the latest population data on the fairy pitta, a bird species found in several Asian countries and classified as vulnerable, was not included in the latest assessment by the International Union for the Conservation of Nature. The reason, again, was that the paper was only published in Chinese.

4 For the new study, Amano's team looked at the entire body of research available on Google Scholar about biodiversity and conservation, starting in the year 2014. Searching with keywords in 16 languages, the researchers found a total of more than 75,000 scientific papers. Of those papers, more than 35 percent were in languages other than English, with Spanish, Portuguese and Chinese topping the list.

5 Even for people who try not to ignore research published in non-English languages, Amano says, difficulties exist. More than half of the non-English papers observed in this study had no English title, abstract or keywords, making them all but invisible to most scientists doing database searches in English. "I think this issue is actually much larger than many people think," Amano says.

6 This problem is a two-way street. Not only does the larger scientific community miss out on research published in non-English languages, but the dominance of English as science's lingua franca makes it more difficult for researchers and policy makers speaking non-English languages to take advantage of science that might help them. For example, of 24 conservation directors in Spain surveyed by Amano and his team, 13 said that a language barrier made their jobs more difficult by limiting their access to information on conservation.

7 It's also worrisome that English has become so prestigious for scientists that many non-English speakers avoid publishing research in their own languages, Amano says. For example, Dutch scientists publish more than 40 papers in English for every 1 article in Dutch, according to a 2012 analysis by the publication Research Trends. The desire to publish in respected English journals is even prompting journals in some countries to decrease or cease publishing in their local languages.

8 Federico Kukso, a MIT Knight Science Journalism fellow who has reported on science in Spanish and English for more than 15 years, says the bias extends beyond how scientists view studies; it also manifests in what science the media chooses to focus on. The Argentina native has previously written about how English-language media tends to ignore the work of Latin American scientists, and especially when these scientists collaborate with American or British scientists.

9 The hegemony of English-language science—and science journalism—has led to the elevation of the work of British and American scientists above that of other nations, Kukso says. He gives an example from earlier this year, when an accomplished

Argentinian paleontologist named Sebastián Apesteguía helped discover a new species of dinosaur. Most English-language media didn't even mention him, instead focusing on his American collaborators.

10 "They don't cover the scientific breakthrough of scientists in Latin America, Asia, Africa, until someone dares to translate it," Kukso says of English-language science journalists. "It's as if non-English science doesn't exist at all." Amano thinks that journals and scientific academies working to include international voices is one of the best solutions to this language gap. He suggests that all major efforts to compile reviews of research include speakers of a variety of languages so that important work isn't overlooked. He also suggests that journals and authors should be pushed to translate summaries of their work into several languages so that it's more easily found by people worldwide. Amano and his collaborators translated a summary of their work into Spanish, Chinese, Portuguese, French and Japanese.

11 Scott Montgomery, a geologist at the University of Washington, agrees that this is an important issue that needs solving. However, when it comes to methodology, Montgomery, who has written extensively on science communication and participated in early peer review process of Amano's paper, thinks that the study "lacks real substance beyond adding to a literature of complaint that has emerged over the past 20 years". The authors took little effort to differentiate between research that was peer-reviewed and research that wasn't in their Google Scholar searches, Montgomery says, making it hard to quantify how much serious research is published in non-English languages. He adds that the authors ignore the historical context of this problem. Just a few decades ago, scientific communication was much harder because there was no dominant lingua franca to publish and share research in, he says.

12 "There were more language barriers, and they were thicker and higher," Montgomery says. While the rise of English as a global and scientific second language does handicap some scientists in other countries, it has also been instrumental in greasing the wheels of communication, he argues. Montgomery is also skeptical of the proposals of Amano and his collaborators to ramp up translation for scientific research. "Scientific translation—which I did part-time for 10 years—is not cheap or fast, and machine translation is a very long way from doing the job, if it ever will," he says.

13 Scientists in all fields would benefit from learning another language, Montgomery says—including native English speakers. But he believes that the best solution to science's language barrier is encouraging scientists worldwide to study English. This may seem unfair to say as a native speaker, he concedes, but as English continues to spread and thrive worldwide, he says it is increasingly necessary. "It is a difficult process, with a rough justice to it," Montgomery says. "But it is profound, human and repeatedly proven." Montgomery and Amano agree on at least one thing: Ignoring language barriers in science is dangerous. "Someone needs to seriously start tackling this issue," Amano says.

Words and Expressions

avian /ˈeɪvɪən/ *adj*.
relating to birds

susceptible /səˈseptɪbl/ *adj*.
likely or liable to be influenced or harmed by a particular thing

veterinary /ˈvetəɪnəri/ *adj*.
connected with caring for the health of animals

dilemma /dɪˈlemə/ *n*.
a situation which makes problems, often one in which you have to make a very difficult choice between things of equal importance

exotic /ɪgˈzɒtɪk/ *adj*.
from or in another country, especially a tropical one; seeming exciting and unusual because it is connected with foreign countries

duplicate /ˈdjuːplɪkeɪt/ *n*.
one of two or more things that are the same in every detail

prompt /prɒmpt/ *v*.
to make sb. decide to do sth.; to cause sth to happen

hegemony /hɪˈdʒeməni/ *n*.
control by one country, organization, etc. over other countries, etc. within a particular group

elevation /ˌelɪˈveɪʃn/ *n*.
the process of sb. getting a higher or more important rank

paleontologist /ˌpæliɒnˈtɒlədʒɪst/ *n*.
a specialist in paleontology

compile /kəmˈpaɪl/ *v*.
to produce a book, list, report, etc. by bringing together different items, articles, songs, etc.

collaborator /kəˈlæbəreɪtə/ *n*.
a person who works with another person to create or produce sth. such as a book

instrumental /ˌɪnstrəˈmentl/ *adj*.
important in making sth. happen

skeptical /ˈskeptɪkl/ *adj*.
having doubts that a claim or statement is true or that sth. will happen

tackle /ˈtækl/ *v*.
to make a determined effort to deal with a difficult problem or situation

I. Reading Comprehension

Choose the best answer to each of the following questions.

1. Why did the author mention the study published in a Chinese journal of veterinary medicine?

    A. Because this study was a great example of success in the development of veterinary medicine in China.

    B. Because the author was an expert in veterinary medicine.

    C. Because the author used it to introduce the topic of the passage.

    D. Because the author took it as an example to show the importance of learning Chinese.

2. What was the dilemma specifically in Paragraph 2?

    A. Language barrier is a major barrier to global science.

    B. It is difficult to translate research papers from Chinese into English.

    C. Language differences can lead to serious international problems.

    D. There is wide gulf between English-language science and any-other-language science.

3. What does "invisible" mean in Paragraph 5?

    A. Non-English papers were neglected by English speaking scientists.

    B. Non-English papers had no impact in the global science.

    C. Non-English papers were generally considered to be of low quality.

    D. Non-English papers couldn't be accessed in English database.

4. Sebastián Apesteguía's experience was taken as an example to show _____.

    A. The hegemony status of English can promote the work of British and American scientists above those of other nations.

    B. Non-native English speaking scientists can also make great achievements.

    C. English-language science can be biased.

    D. The hegemony status of English bring injustice in science.

5. Which of the following is NOT a suggested solution to the language problem in the global science?

    A. Compiling reviews of researches of a variety of languages.

    B. Requiring peer review for all research papers.

    C. Translating summaries of research works into several languages.

    D. Encouraging scientists worldwide to study English.

II. Vocabulary

Task 1 *Fill in the blanks of the following sentences with the words or expressions given in the box below. Change the forms where necessary.*

susceptible	skeptical	hegemony	conservation	solution
subtype	strain	veterinary	profound	two-way street
tackle	avian	exotic	compile	collaborator

1. In total, about 30 schools and colleges from around the region have joined together to _____ a comprehensive booklet of what is available.

2. The availability of grants in contributing towards the repairs and _____ of historic buildings has been very significant.

3. The company is dedicated to providing personalized student lending _____ to schools and students to increase access to education.

4. Not only does he need to convince a _____ market, he also has to reach an increasingly disillusioned customer.

5. The lack of knowledge about AIDS and venereal diseases generally makes this group particularly _____ to infection.

6. The workshop left me in a _____ state of wonder at the subtlety and simplicity of this healing approach.

7. For some people, US _____ was a specific phase of capitalist expansion in the post-war era.

8. You want to make sure your pet is as healthy as can be and part of dog ownership is to provide your dog with excellent _____ care.

9. It has been less clearly understood that this relationship may well be a _____ , with causation possibly working in the opposite direction as well.

10. This bird was an escapee of some manner of _____ imprisonment, maybe a zoo.

11. Their extensive network of facilities, efficient administration and commitment to serving the poor, he thought, would make them ideal _____ .

12. I _____ him about how anyone could live amidst so much poverty.

13. It remains a major agricultural problem, especially for potato farmers who have been breeding resistant _____ .

14. The _____ creature, which originates from Central and South America, is probably an escaped pet.

15. Winter vomiting is due to infection with _____ of the genus Norwalk-like virus,

a term that is now preferred to small round structured virus.

(Task 2) *Under each of the following boxes there are several groups of sentences. In each sentence a common word or expression is missing. Find it out from the corresponding box according to the meaning and structure of the sentences. The forms of the words and expressions may change in the sentences.*

dilemma	instrumental	duplicate	elevation

Group 1

1. The sedative and analgesic effects are caused by the stimulation of central alpha-2 adrenoceptors, while the stimulation of peripheral alpha-2 adrenoceptors causes peripheral vasoconstriction resulting in a transitory blood pressure _____ and bradycardia.

2. An _____ in intracellular Ca^{2+} increases the activity of CaN, which dephosphorylates the NFAT molecule and allows its import into the nucleus.

3. Group 2 contained 15(31%) cases with low to intermediate _____ of cyclin D1 mRNA and no evidence of the t(11;14) translocation.

Answer: _____

Group 2

1. The inflammatory response that occurs in the CNS during EAE was _____ in up-regulating Ag presentation, as CNS APCs isolated from healthy mice were relatively inefficient at presenting Ag directly ex vivo.

2. We would like to thank Prof. David Billington and Dr. Dan Rathbone for kindly providing the _____ facilities of MS, FTIR and NMR.

3. This finding illustrates that combinations of polymorphic genes may act in concert in the pathogenesis of SLE, a concept that may be _____ in the analysis of the genetics of SLE as well as providing hypotheses for pathways in the pathogenesis.

Answer: _____

Group 3

1. The classic _____ of the management of postinfarction ventricular septal defect (PIVSD) is the timing of intervention: most of the patients require an emergent repair to improve hemodynamics, while intentional deferment of intervention allows reducing the risk of residual shunt through organization and fibrosis of the frail infarct tissue.

2. This leads radiologists to the _____ of balancing sensitivity and specificity.

3. Notwithstanding unprecedented volume of investigations on the H. pylori infection worldwide，its effective eradication remains as a _____ .

Answer：_____

Group 4

1. All samples were prepared in _____ .

2. Each assay was performed in _____ , and at least five fields were counted randomly to determine the number of adherent cells.

3. All assays presented here were performed at least three times by _____

Answer：_____

| overlooked | extensively | effort | prompt |

Group 5

1. Fast track endoscopy has been introduced to _____ diagnosis for patients with alarm symptoms that could be indicative of upper GI cancer.

2. The present studies should _____ further research to study genes induced by IFN- and Mtb that are relevant to the pathophysiology of tuberculosis.

3. The initial treatment of unstable UGIB in our ED includes resuscitation with crystalloid and blood transfusions，intravenous vasopressin，and _____ consultation with a specialist.

Answer：_____

Group 6

1. In an effort to achieve these goals，intraocular lens（IOL）materials and designs have been studied _____ , and considerable attention has been directed to improving the optical quality provided by IOLs.

2. Diabetes is an _____ investigated disease，characterized by elevated serum glucose，which might result in internal organ damage when not carefully controlled.

3. Then，the NK cells were _____ washed in phosphate-buffered saline（PBS），fixed and the percentage of positive cells was analyzed with fluorescence activated cell sorting.

Answer：_____

Group 7

1. One clinically important，but often _____ , cardiovascular consequence is that diabetic and obese patients have increased requirements for surgical treatments.

2. Given that most of those studies were performed with critically ill patients with the purpose of controlling fever, the researchers could have _____ the differences that may exist between the causes of fever.

3. Emergency care practitioners and health-care professionals often _____ the importance of greeting each other.

Answer: _____

Group 8

1. In adults, hypotension and symptoms of orthostatic intolerance are seen in individuals with increased inspiratory _____ during sleep.

2. Considerable _____ has been mounted towards developing strategies for generating transplantable HSCs from alternative cell types, such as pluripotent (ES/iPS) stem cells.

3. In view of this, there has been a concerted _____ to develop a new and improved vaccine against TB.

Answer: _____

III. Cloze

Fill in each of the following blanks with the most appropriate word from each of the four choices given.

In the late twentieth century, English became the "lingua franca" of science. Over 80% of peer-reviewed journals across all scientific disciplines in the SCOPUS database are written in English. Similarly, data from across all areas of healthcare indicate that 80–90% of articles are published in English. The __1__ of English in scientific publications means that __2__ in English enables researchers, clinicians and other users of research to capitalize on research findings to a greater extent. This may explain why a global survey found that a country's English proficiency __3__ with its level of innovation.

The most recent data show that approximately 20% of the world's working age population speaks English and less than 5% have English as their first language. An evaluation of global internet utilization __4__ that English accounts for 25% of usage, followed by Chinese (19%), Spanish (8%), and Arabic (5%).

Clinicians, policy makers, educators, and researchers may encounter difficulty in identifying and reading high-quality research if they are not able to __5__ resources in their native language. Recent surveys of Brazilian physical therapists have found that whilst they are motivated to __6__ research into their clinical practice, the predominance of resources in English appears to be a __7__ as resources in Portuguese are accessed preferentially. This language barrier could result in unnecessary __8__ of research, as well as introducing bias into clinical decision-making.

The __9__ between the proportion of articles published in English (80-90%) and the global proficiency in the English language (20-25%) __10__ the need for strategies to enable equitable access to research. Advances in machine learning capabilities have led to the development of online translation tools, but the accuracy of machine translations may be __11__ to support clinical decision-making. Translation issues include __12__ with finding equivalent vocabulary and working with an entirely different syntax, as well as difficulty displaying the language script. Translating sections of text out of context may fail to __13__ a reliable translation, which may be __14__ in understanding the research. Professional translation services would address these issues, but creates a financial barrier for researchers.

To help reduce the language barrier to consuming research, providers of bibliographic databases have started using translation and __15__ strategies. For example, the Cumulative Index of Nursing and Allied Health Literature (CINAHL) database allows users to search for articles using any of 24 different languages. Ovid Technologies provide natural language search interfaces in seven languages (English, French, German, Spanish, Chinese, Japanese, Korean). PubMed is developing multilingual search engine interfaces, as well as allowing users to search for transliterated titles using English characters.

1. A. priority   B. predominance   C. preoccupation   D. preference
2. A. efficiency   B. sufficiency   C. proficiency   D. adequacy
3. A. correlates   B. relates   C. correspond   D. combine
4. A. relates   B. conveys   C. prevails   D. reveals
5. A. access   B. deliver   C. accumulate   D. facilitate
6. A. conduct   B. incorporate   C. carry   D. perform
7. A. choice   B. barrier   C. chance   D. problem
8. A. procedures   B. cost   C. burden   D. duplication
9. A. misconception   B. mismatch   C. misunderstanding   D. misfortune
10. A. results in   B. leads to   C. points to   D. relies on
11. A. insufficient   B. inappropriate   C. adequate   D. sufficient
12. A. processes   B. difficulty   C. features   D. requirements
13. A. translate   B. revise   C. yield   D. edit
14. A. unnecessary   B. reliable   C. accountable   D. critical
15. A. multi-language B. international   C. cooperative   D. sustainable

IV. Discussion and Presentation

Answer the following questions on the basis of your reading.

1. Who do you agree with more? Montgomery or Amano?

2. Is hegemony of English and diversity of language a barrier or contributor to the development of global science?

3. As a non-native English speaker, what is your solution to the language barrier confronted by the global science?

V. Translation

Translate the following sentences into English.

1. 信息和通信技术的迅速发展使翻译朝着让用户获得更多信息、提供更多信得过产品的方向迈出了新的一步。

2. 继 2003 年报告猪感染 H5N1 型病毒和 2005 年至 2006 年报告家禽市场出现该病毒的高致病性禽流感之后，我们分别于 2004 年和 2007 年对福建省养猪场猪群开展了禽流感病毒血清阳性率的调查。

3. 根据生产商的说明进行 H1N1 和 H3N2 的 ELISA 试验，并使用生产商提供的公式将得到的光密度值转换为 S/P 值。

4. 应该注意的是，H5 和 H9 的 HI 试验方法、抗原和阳性血清均与李＊＊等人（2004 年）研究中的方法、抗原和阳性血清相同，并且所有试验均在血清样本收集后不久进行。

5. 我们分别于 2004 年和 2007 年在被调查猪群中采集了 499 份和 908 份血清样本，做了流感病毒感染的血清学检测。

VI. Further Readings

1. Serological Surveillance of Influenza: A Virus Infection in Fujian

2. Languages Are Still a Major Barrier to Global Science

3. Machine Translation as an Academic Writing Aid for Medical Practitioners

Part II : Academic Development

I. Translating Medical Texts

Read the following sample abstract and put the underlined part into English.

【摘要】猪是禽流感病毒"禽-猪-人"传播链中重要的中间宿主,了解猪流感的疫情动态将为动物流感及人流感的疾病预测及防治提供重要依据。1999~2001 年间进行的血清学和病毒学监测发现我国猪群存在大范围的 H1 和 H3 亚型猪流感感染(李海燕等,2002)。2002~2003 年,我们进一步对来自全国 14 个省市的 1936 份血清进行了 H9 亚型猪流感的检测,同时在广东、福建等省进行了 H5 亚型猪流感的检测。2002 年辽宁、广东、山东及重庆猪血清中出现 H9 亚型流感抗体,阳性率分别为 7.3%、6.8%、5.1%和 1.6%。2003 年采集的猪血清 H9 亚型流感抗体均为阴性,同时发现广东、福建两省 2003 年出现 H5 亚型流感阳性猪群,阳性率分别为 4.7%和 8.2%。从 2001~2003 年收集和送检的样品中分离鉴定了 6 株 H9N2 亚型和 2 株 H5N1 亚型猪流感病毒,部分序列分析发现 H9 和 H5 亚型猪流感病毒均与我国分离的禽流感病毒高度同源。本研究进一步确证了我国猪群中存在 H9N2 亚型流感病毒,并且首次发现我国猪群已出现 H5N1 亚型流感病毒,为人类流感及动物流感的防治敲响了警钟。对这两个亚型流感病毒所具有的公共卫生和兽医公共卫生危害性应予以高度重视。①

> **Translation & Writing Skills: Passive Voice vs Active Voice**

English language generally tends to use more passive voice than Chinese. Passive voice is frequently used in informative texts rather than imaginative writing, notably in objective, non-personal scientific articles and news items. This feature is actually closely related to the impersonal subject of English sentences since the passive voice allows one to express ideas without attributing them to a specific individual source. However, it does not mean passive voice is better than active voice or the other way around. It is wise to learn which voice should be used in particular cases.

Active voice can be employed to report original research, promote and emphasise a finding, demonstrate how your work improves on the work of others and how innovative and unique the research is. Examples are as follows:

---

① 选自《中国预防兽医学报》2004 年第 1 期,1-6 页。作者:李海燕,于康震,杨焕良,辛晓光,陈君彦,赵普,毕英佐,陈化兰。

Example 1：PS 不仅能够有效地诱导 BALB/C 和 Tg 小鼠（转基因小鼠）的体液免疫，还能抑制 Tg 小鼠 HbsAg 的产生。

PS is effective to elicit a positive humor immune response in BALB/C mice. PS can also stimulate an immune response in Tg mice，which seems to be responsible for the disappearance of HbsAg.

Example 2：对 45 例肝硬化门静脉高压患者分别应用乌拉地尔（N＝15）和西咪替丁（n＝20）和 0.9%氯化钠盐水（n＝10）后，观察其肝静脉楔入压（WHVP）、肝静脉压力梯度（HVPG）及全身血流动力学的影响。

We observed the effects of urapidil（urapidil HCl，n＝15），cimetidine（n＝20）and placebo（0.9% sodium chloride，n＝10）on wedeged haptic venous pressure （WHVP），hepatic venous pressure gradient（HVPG）and systemic homodynamics.

Example 3：将合并有至少一个肾以外的器官衰竭或脓毒血症的急性肾损伤危重患者随机分配到强化或非强化肾替代治疗组。

We randomly assigned critically ill patients with acute kidney injury and failure of at least one normal organ or sepsis to receive intensive or less intensive renal-replacement therapy.

Passive voice is preferred when who does something is less important than the recipient of the action or when it doesn't matter who performed the action. It is effective at describing methods and procedures and adds formality to the text. It is also used when the author wishes to remain neutral. It takes the focus off the subject or the person carrying out the action and puts attention onto the way something has been carried out.

Examples：

Example 4：采用生化法、放射免疫法、荧光分析法及逆转录-聚合酶链反应技术等进行研究。

Techniques including biochemistry，radioimmunoassay，fiuoroassays and Reverse Transcription-polymerase chain reaction（RT-PCR）were used in this study.

Example 5：30 例非糖尿病常规血液透析患者随机分成硝苯地平组、罗钙全组和安慰剂组。

30 non-diabetic uremic patients undergoing maintenance hemodialysis were divided into nifedipine group，calcitriol group and placebo group.

Example 6：没有发现支持服用萘普森可以降低心肌梗死发生率的证据。

No evidence was found to support a reduction in risk of myocardial infarction associated with the current use of naproxen.

II. Writing Medical Papers in English

How to Write a Conclusion for a Research Paper
By Christopher Taylor

The conclusion of a research paper needs to summarize the content and purpose of the paper without seeming too wooden or dry. Every basic conclusion must share several key elements，but there are also several tactics you can play around with to craft a more effective conclusion and several you should avoid to prevent yourself from weakening your paper's conclusion. Here are some writing tips to keep in mind when creating a conclusion for your next research paper.

Writing a Basic Conclusion

1. Restate the topic. You should briefly restate the topic as well as explaining why it is important.

- Do not spend a great amount of time or space restating your topic.
- A good research paper will make the importance of your topic apparent，so you do not need to write an elaborate defense of your topic in the conclusion.
- Usually a single sentence is all you need to restate your topic.
- An example would be if you were writing a paper on the epidemiology of an infectious disease，you might say something like "Tuberculosis is a widespread infectious disease that affects millions of people worldwide every year."
- Yet another example from the humanities would be a paper about the Italian Renaissance："The Italian Renaissance was an explosion of art and ideas centered around artists，writers，and thinkers in Florence."

2. Restate your thesis. Aside from the topic，you should also restate or rephrase your thesis statement.

- A thesis is a narrowed，focused view on the topic at hand.
- This statement should be rephrased from the thesis you included in your introduction. It should not be identical or too similar to the sentence you originally used.
- Try re-wording your thesis statement in a way that complements your summary of

the topic of your paper in your first sentence of your conclusion.

- An example of a good thesis statement, going back to the paper on tuberculosis, would be "*Tuberculosis is a widespread disease that affects millions of people worldwide every year. Due to the alarming rate of the spread of tuberculosis, particularly in poor countries, medical professionals are implementing new strategies for the diagnosis, treatment, and containment of this disease.*"

3. Briefly summarize your main points. Essentially, you need to remind your readers what you told them in the body of the paper.

- A good way to go about this is to re-read the topic sentence of each major paragraph or section in the body of your paper.
- Find a way to briefly restate each point mentioned in each topic sentence in your conclusion. Do not repeat any of the supporting details used within your body paragraphs.
- Under most circumstances, you should avoid writing new information in your conclusion. This is especially true if the information is vital to the argument or research presented in your paper.
- For example, in the TB paper you could summarize the information. "*Tuberculosis is a widespread disease that affects millions of people worldwide. Due to the alarming rate of the spread of tuberculosis, particularly in poor countries, medical professionals are implementing new strategies for the diagnosis, treatment, and containment of this disease. In developing countries, such as those in Africa and Southeast Asia, the rate of TB infections is soaring. Crowded conditions, poor sanitation, and lack of access to medical care are all compounding factors in the spread of the disease. Medical experts, such as those from the World Health Organization are now starting campaigns to go into communities in developing countries and provide diagnostic testing and treatments. However, the treatments for TB are very harsh and have many side effects. This leads to patient non-compliance and spread of multi-drug resistant strains of the disease.*"

4. Add the points up. If your paper proceeds in an inductive manner and you have not fully explained the significance of your points yet, you need to do so in your conclusion.

- Note that this is not needed for all research papers.
- If you already fully explained what the points in your paper mean or why they are significant, you do not need to go into them in much detail in your conclusion. Simply restating your thesis or the significance of your topic should

suffice.

- It is always best practice to address important issues and fully explain your points in the body of your paper. The point of a conclusion to a research paper is to summarize your argument for the reader and, perhaps, to call the reader to action if needed.

5. Make a call to action when appropriate. If and when needed, you can state to your readers that there is a need for further research on your paper's topic.

- Note that a call for action is not essential to all conclusions. A research paper on literary criticism, for instance, is less likely to need a call for action than a paper on the effect that television has on toddlers and young children.
- A paper that is more likely to call readers to action is one that addresses a public or scientific need. Let's go back to our example of tuberculosis. This is a very serious disease that is spreading quickly and with antibiotic-resistant forms.
- A call to action in this research paper would be a follow-up statement that might be along the lines of *"Despite new efforts to diagnose and contain the disease, more research is needed to develop new antibiotics that will treat the most resistant strains of tuberculosis and ease the side effects of current treatments"*.

6. Answer the "so what" question. The conclusion of a paper is your opportunity to explain the broader context of the issue you have been discussing. It is also a place to help readers understand why the topic of your paper truly matters. You should use the conclusion to answer the "so what" question because the significance of your topic may not be obvious to readers. For example, if you are writing a history paper, then you might discuss how the historical topic you discussed matters today. If you are writing about a foreign country, then you might use the conclusion to discuss how the information you shared may help readers understand their own country.

参考文献

［1］Aniruddha Mitra，James Thomas Bang，Arnab Biswas. Gender Equality and Economic Growth：Is it Equality of Opportunity or Equality of Outcomes? ［J］. Feminist Economics，2015(1)：1-38.

［2］Anne Marie Helmenstine. How to Write an Abstract for a Scientific Paper ［OL］. ［2019-06-26］https：//www. thoughtco. com/writing-an-abstract-for-a-scientific-paper-609106.

［3］Bowker Lynne，Ciro Jairo-Buitrago. Machine Translation and Global Research：Towards Improved Machine Translation Literacy in the Scholarly Community ［M］. Bingley：Emerald Publishing Ltd，2019.

［4］Grace Fleming. Finding Statistics and Data for Research Papers ［OL］. ［2020-01-29］https：//www. thoughtco. com/finding-statistics-for-research-papers-1857284.

［5］Haavi Morreim. Research versus Innovation：Real Differences ［J］. The American Journal of Bioethics，2005(2)：42-43.

［6］Hart Steve. Writing in English for the Medical Sciences ［M］. Florida：CRC Press，2016.

［7］Hutchinson T. & Waters. English for Specific Purposes—A Learning-Centred Approach ［M］. New York：Cambridge University Press，1987.

［8］Kenneth Beare. Linking Your Ideas in English with Discourse Markers ［OL］. ［2018-04-05］https：//www. thoughtco. com/discourse-markers-linking-your-ideas-1208952.

［9］Kenneth Beare. Passive Voice Usage and Examples for ESL/EFL (OL). ［2019-01-05］https：//www. thoughtco. com/passive-voice-in-english-grammar-1211144.

［10］Lucas Nunes Vieira，Minako O'Hagan，Carol O'Sullivan. Understanding the Societal Impacts of Machine Translation：A Critical Review of the Literature on

Medical and Legal Use Cases [J]. Information，Communication & Society，2020，24(11)：1-18.

[11] Mehmet Burcu，Cyntia B. Manzano-Salgado，Anne M. Butler，Jennifer B. Christian. A Framework for Extension Studies Using Real-World Data to Examine Long-Term Safety and Effectiveness [J/OL]. Therapeutic Innovation & Regulatory Science，2021（6）：1 - 8. https：//doi. org/10. 1007/s43441-021-00322-8.

[12] Montalt Vicent-&-González-Davies-Maria. Medical Translation Step by Step：Learning by Drafting [M]. New York：Taylor and Francis，2014.

[13] Moore P.J. Murphy P. Pascucci L. & Sustenance S. Machine Translation for EFL [J]. Relay Journal，2019,2(1)：228-235.

[14] Orkan Okan，Ullrich Bauer，Diane Levin-Zamir，Paulo Pinheiro and Kristine Sorensen. International Handbook Of Health Literacy [M]. Bristol：Policy Press，2019

[15] Taylor Robert-B. Medical Writing：A Guide for Clinicians，Educators，and Researchers [M]. Switzerland：Springer International Publishing，2018.

[16] Wallwork Adrian. English for Writing Research Papers [M]. New York：Springer，2011.

[17] 陈兴怡,翟绍果.中国共产党百年卫生健康治理的历史变迁、政策逻辑与路径方向[J].西北大学学报(哲学社会科学版),2021(7)：86-94.

[18] 从丛."中国文化失语"：我国英语教学的缺陷[N].光明日报.2019-10-19.

[19] 费太安.健康中国百年求索——党领导下的我国医疗卫生事业发展历程及经验[J].管理世界,2021(11)：26-40.

[20] 巩高,黄文华,曹石,等.人工智能在医学的应用研究进展[J].中国医学物理学杂志,2021(8)：1044-1047.

[21] 李海燕,于康震,杨焕良,等.中国猪源 H5N1 和 H9N2 亚型流感病毒的分离鉴定[J].中国预防兽医学报,2004(1)：1-6.

[22] 李明,苏伟,周婷,等.临床实习压力对医学生心理健康影响的调查[J].中国健康心理学杂志,2017(4)：595-598.

[23] 李宛亭,乔佳慧,孟令全,等.真实世界数据存在的问题与质量提升对策研究[J].中国新药杂志,2021(13)：1160-1163.

[24] 司显柱.试论我国高校英语教学中的意识形态[J].语言教育,2018,6(2)：2-4,8.

[25] 苏孟宇,王真,张玉玺,等.居家安宁疗护对晚期癌症患者生活质量和情绪影响的 Meta 分析[J].中华护理杂志,2021(8)：1249-1255.

[26] 陶应时,罗成翼.人类胚胎基因编辑的伦理悖论及其化解之道[J].自然辩证法通讯,2018(2)：85-91.

［27］王晶,杨小科.中国农村基层医疗卫生改革的制度选择与发展反思［J］.东北师大学报
（哲学社会科学版）,2014(6)：68-73.

［28］魏清光.中国文学"走出去"：现状、问题及对策［J］.当代文坛,2015(1)：155-159.

［29］吴月齐.试论高校推进"课程思政"的三个着力点［J］.学校党建与思想教育,2018(1)：
67-69.

［30］夏文红,何芳.大学英语"课程思政"的使命担当［J］.人民论坛,2019(30)：108-109.

［31］闫积存.改良流程化护理干预在急诊外科中的运用观察［J］.甘肃科技,2021(17)：
148-150.

［32］杨萌,石旭雯.医疗机器人伦理设计进路初探［J］.中国医学伦理学,2020(7)：
873-878.

［33］姚宏文,石琦,李英华.我国城乡居民健康素养现状及对策［J］.人口研究,2016(2)：
88-97.

［34］周晓姗,陈万明.脑血管病全脑血管造影和介入治疗的临床护理研究［J］.智慧健康,
2021(7)：168-170.